Molar Pregnancy
70+ Questions Answered

Lydia Kariuki

Molar Pregnancy
Copyright © 2018

ISBN: 9781977036483

Warning and Disclaimer
Every effort has been made to make this book as accurate as possible. However, no warranty or fitness is implied. The information provided is on an "as-is" basis. The author and the publisher shall have no liability or responsibility to any person or entity with respect to any loss or damages that arise from the information in this book.

Publisher Contact
Skinny Bottle Publishing
books@skinnybottle.com

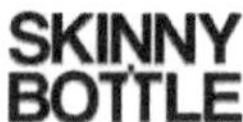

Introduction

Akin to wine, age is a trusted friend.

In my clinical nursing experience, I have acquired critical soft skills through time and perseverance; these skills cannot be acquired from medical textbooks or sheer intelligence. But I have also learned how to make up for a lack of eons of experience by reading widely and having deep conversations with my patients. After all, it is only the patient who can educate you on their true symptoms and feelings at any one point in time. The patient is the best textbook of any one condition. They are the true professors.

The year is 2008 and I am working as a nurse intern in a local government hospital in Mombasa, Kenya. This is my third rotation and I am still very eager to impress! I am not yet stuck up in routines, procedures, and deliverables. Every case is almost a first one and makes a profound impression on my heart. Every evening I go home pondering cases and "feeling" with the patient. This period also involves a lot of reading for two reasons; every case is new, and I need to gain knowledge on it and two, I have a licensing exam to sit for at the end of all the rotations.

Obgyn ward rotation starts

It is a normal Wednesday morning when I start this rotation. After a short walk around to familiarize myself with the ward set up, I am all set for work. The staffs seem friendly but are not eager to engage me much. Perhaps too tired with overzealous interns like myself who think they can "change the world" with their sheer zeal and determination, the assumption being that whatever is being done presently is wanting. Thankfully, I have already done two other rotations so I have mastered techniques of getting the senior staff to like you and be of help. I quickly locate the duty roster and find the team that I have been assigned to work with during my one-month rotation in this ward. It is the green team and I find out that the outgoing staff is handing over to the new team. I quickly join them. I listen in and try to be of as much help as I can. In the end, the team in charge asks my name. Woo-hoo! I think I am on track.

The third patient on my team happens to be a molar pregnancy patient who is being prepped for her second round of chemotherapy. Actually, the case is persistent gestational trophoblastic disease. I scratch my head trying to recall what this was and how it presented, I then give up and resort to my phone to search. Clearly, I did not meet a "live case" during my training at the national referral hospital. Else, I would recall.

After I have updated my knowledge, I approach the nurse attending to the patient and ask how I can be of help. She turns to me and asks for how long I have been in the ward. Then I think she places me as the new intern who was present for the early morning round. She then goes ahead to offer, "do nothing, just stay here and watch."

Amina, the patient, seems to be the cool, calm and collected kind. She is neither anxious nor distraught. This is her second cycle. I also notice that there is no one with her, I mean family or friend. When the nurse leaves briefly, I decide to engage her and offer comfort. Then it hits me, I don't really know what to say. Has she lost a baby? What exactly should I say?

Then I notice something, she has some baby clothes in her baby bag which she is still carrying around. Hmm, it is a newborn sweater. I am certain that it cannot be for another child, it must have been intended for this child who no longer is. Amina is still walking around with this sweater, perhaps for memory's sake? I am not sure.

Soon, the nurse is back, and the procedure begins. I engage myself in making sure that Amina is comfortable and the nurse, my colleague, is assisted in every possible way. When it is done, Amina is too tired, and I ensure that she rests immediately. She will be leaving for home tomorrow if all goes as planned.

Before the end of my shift, I peruse through all patient files and learn that there are three patients admitted with molar pregnancy-related conditions. One with a fresh molar diagnosis set for an ERCP while the other two with persistent GTDs.

The next time I am on shift, all three patients are not there but there is a new patient with a molar pregnancy. I get the privilege to assist in the ERCP procedure. During the procedure, the silence in the room is deafening. And my mind is racing trying to find appropriate words. What do you say after the procedure? "Mum, we are done?" Quite confusing isn't it. To fill up the emptiness, the nurse quickly goes on to give instructions on follow up visits, contraception, and the likes. All this time, the patient remains silent, asking no question.

This stirs something in me, but still, I don't feel equipped enough to engage with the patient at a deep level. And from what I sense, no one around me does. A nurse would occasionally throw a kind comment here and there like, "don't you worry, you will get another baby soon" but I could tell that it hardly broke through to the patient's emotions. I realized that my medical knowledge fell short in this one vital area. And nothing can quite make up for a real-life experience, being there with the patient, feeling with them and providing deep answers to questions that they are struggling to ask.

I took a dive into the deep end. By the end of the one month, not only was I equipped medically to walk the patient through the journey from diagnosis to treatment to life after a molar pregnancy, but I was also able to help them deal with significant fears surrounding a molar pregnancy diagnosis.

Over time, I have learned that it is imperative for patients to bring out their deep questions and find answers to them to be able to achieve complete healing.

There is a lot of mystery surrounding molar pregnancies, perhaps due to the low incidence. Adequate awareness has not been created. I have been able to do better as an informed nurse offering care to victims of molar pregnancies. Also, I have learned that patients who speak more openly and ask questions heal faster and are able to move on faster. That's why I set out to compile my experience, research, and consultations into this short volume of 70 plus questions on molar pregnancy for patients, their partners and their caregivers. Welcome aboard!

Chapter One

MOLAR PREGNANCY INCIDENCE AND STATISTICS

In the US, the incidence of molar pregnancy is 1 in every 1000 women. The incidence is slightly higher in Southeast Asia, that is eight times higher! Mexico, the Philippines, and African women also have a higher incidence than women in the US. Generally, white women living in the US have the lowest incidence of molar pregnancy.

That said, any woman of childbearing age can get a molar pregnancy irrespective of geographical location or race. Many factors such as age, menstrual cycle irregularities, and genetic factors can predispose one to a molar pregnancy. It is good for every woman of childbearing age to be acquainted with the relevant information about this condition.

A shortcoming of the above statistics is inadequate follow-up after a miscarriage, especially in developing nations. When a woman miscarries, sometimes she is not followed up as should be. She may go home assuming that she had a normal miscarriage, but what actually happened is that she had a molar pregnancy which ended up as a miscarriage. Miscarriages happen for a variety of reasons, one of them is a molar pregnancy. A molar pregnancy mimics a normal pregnancy in so many ways that it can be assumed to be a normal pregnancy unless put under greater scrutiny such as scans, Hcg tests and careful examination of the products of conception. It takes the eye and skill of an expert to tell the difference between the two, especially in the early days. It is only in the event of a persistent molar pregnancy, that symptoms of pregnancy will not diminish therefore alerting the patient that something may be wrong. But even in this case, some women have mistaken this to be a consequent pregnancy only to discover too late that it was a case of persistent gestational trophoblastic disease.

The other challenge posed in collecting data is the apprehension surrounding molar pregnancies. The issue of reproduction touches to the core of femininity. A woman needs to be able to bear children for the continuity of humanity. When this capability is challenged in any way, shame creeps in and we talk about it in hushed tones. When a molar pregnancy happens, we prefer to assume that nothing big ever happened and it was for the best, or there was no child in the first place and so forth. By so doing, we entrench the shame and apprehension surrounding molar pregnancy.

Lastly, there isn't enough awareness created about molar pregnancy. Health facilities and health care providers are not primed to spot and offer adequate support for molar pregnancy victims. This is especially true in developing nations. Many times, I have seen and read about patients who ask, "Why was this not obvious to my doctor or nurse?" This is after they have researched widely on molar pregnancy after their diagnosis and they discover that they had some obvious signs pointing towards a molar pregnancy diagnosis.

That said, every woman deserves to be informed and educated about molar pregnancy. If not personally affected, perhaps a sister, colleague or friend can get affected. In that case, she will be a caregiver who needs to offer support to the affected woman. The other role every woman should play is to be an ambassador of victims of molar pregnancy. Molar pregnancy is a reality affecting women of every nation and can happen to any of us. The better equipped we are as a team to combat it, the better for us all.

A success story; Mary and Mark

Mary and Mark, not their actual names, are a pair that has stuck together through the diagnosis and treatment of molar pregnancy and have lived to tell their story that inspires hope and faith!

Back in 2012, Mary was working as a clerk in a government office while Mark had a managerial position in a different department of the same government ministry.

Back at home, the formidable pair had four children aged between 1.5 and 7. That is the real definition of having a house full, with diapers, car seats, strollers and food leftovers in tiny cups and plates strewn all over the place. They rarely had "spare time" to sit and relax as a couple. Thankfully, they could see each other in between tasks in the office or at lunch break. But even then, they preferred to grab a nap in the back of their Nissan caravan.

This particular Monday, Mary was a bit too exhausted to do anything at work. She contemplated taking yet another sick off to go home and rest, but as she walked past the office kitchen to the locker room to collect her bag, something struck her. She was nauseous at the aroma of eggs that had saturated the air in the kitchen. Coming to think of it, she had skipped breakfast the last three mornings because she could not stand the smell of bacon, or eggs, or even buttered toast. What!

The ground beneath her began to spin so fast that she thought she was going to fall, she leaned back against the wall for support. As soon as she had rested enough to gain control of her gait, she rushed for her bag and sprinted to her car and drove off to the nearest chemist. All the way she was mumbling to herself that it could not have happened. The more she thought about it, the more scared she got, she could not recall when she had her menses last!

It took her fifteen minutes to dash from the office to the chemist, to her house and into the loo, record time! Then it happened, the two red lines appeared! She just sank to the floor not even having the energy to call her hubby.

When Mark came home that evening, he was already aware that Mary had taken early leave from work, again. He found the usual mess in the house but Mary was nowhere to be seen. He walked to the bedroom where he found Mary and toddler Kaylen asleep in bed together. But just before he began to make noise about the co-sleeping, he saw the two strips beside the bed. Needless to say, the pair was least prepared for another addition to the sextet.

After absorbing in the shock, the pair accepted their fate and joked that this was a bonus child and so must be a real surprise from heaven. They slept after scheduling a doctor's appointment that Friday.

Friday comes and after dropping the kids at school, they find themselves at the obgyns waiting bay, again. From the dates, it turns out that Mary is already three months pregnant!

In the doctor's office, the doctor asks Mary a battery of routine questions, but he seems dissatisfied with her answers. He then performs a routine examination, and then lastly, he concludes that he needs to do a scan.

It is when doing the scan that he drops the news like a bombshell, "Mary, what you have is a molar pregnancy"

Mary looked at the doctor pretending to comprehend what he meant but at the back of her mind, she was struggling to remember where she had heard that word and what it meant. At first, molar tooth came to her mind, but she laughed it off. Then she looked at Mark and read his face, it then hit her. It is Mark's cousin who had a molar pregnancy back in 2010!

Now she knew what it meant, they were not going to have another baby, after all. So, were they to give each a pat on the back and say hooray! Or were they to break down and cry for their lost child? The silence in the room was deafening as the medics stared at this condensed pair. It was up to them to give the lead on the emotions that the team was to adapt. For the pair, one word described their feelings, "perplexed!"

ERCP

All four of Mary's previous pregnancies had been SVDs (spontaneous vertex deliveries) meaning vaginal births. So, she was kinder used to being put in the birth position with legs suspended midair and nurses rubbing your head as they wipe streaks of sweat from your forehead. However, two things were visibly missing today, the sweat and the shrieking cry that tears through the roof once the baby is out. But this time around, Mary was prepared to take the lead. As soon as the procedure was done, she profusely thanked the nurses and made a light joke that four babies should be enough for any sane couple. Mark laughed uncomfortably, and the nurse gave an awkward smile and mumbled something incomprehensible. The room then retreated to the awkward silence. Honestly, Mary felt or thought that she felt okay at this point. Perhaps she was only guilty of feeling nothing when the nurse tried to offer her some Kleenex and later some contacts of a therapist that helped women deal with molar pregnancy associated depression.

The drive back home was silent as both Mary and Mark tried to process what had just transpired. Mark seemed more affected by the event, perhaps having witnessed something similar with his cousin two years ago. He even felt that he needed to see a therapist to process the loss, but he would be glad if Mary was willing to accompany him. Mary, on the other hand, didn't feel the same, she was okay. And anyway, they both had full-time jobs and four budding kids to keep them occupied 2/4/7. Where do you fit in therapy time in this overstretched schedule?

Hcg monitoring for six months

The next six months was a roller coaster for this budding family as they struggled with different emotions surrounding the diagnosis of a molar pregnancy. At first, Mark went in to see a therapist but dropped out after a single session as Mary nagged him to forget the incidence and move on. On the contrary, Mary tried to justify her attitude by talking to friends who were first astounded that she could have fallen pregnant again after having vowed to get the knot after her fourth baby. After the astonishment came the hurtful consolation that the baby was deformed so it was better that it did not survive. All this came from genuine hearts that wanted to give her comfort, but they were just so misinformed that every time Mary shared this with anyone, it left her feeling ten times worse than she previously was.

Within no time, Mary became an emotional wreck and resorted to closet drinking to numb her feelings shut out the questions. Then the haunt began. She would be in bed at night then she would hear the cry of her baby. One night she woke up screaming that she wanted to go to the hospital to collect her baby. She could swear that she had seen the nurse stash her baby away in a locker and she knew that the nurse wanted to sell her baby. Mark managed to put her back to sleep with some meds. But early the next morning, they both began therapy, which they did for four consecutive months. As they say, it was the best decision they ever made, especially since it prepared them for what lay ahead of them. Without therapy, they would have crumbled.

As this was happening, Mary's Hcg levels were being monitored monthly. As so much was going on in her life emotionally, she never paid attention to the reports. Three months into the monitoring, she received a call from her doctor asking her to prepare for an admission for chemotherapy.

What! How does one person get so unlucky? She was alone in the house that day as granny had picked the kids for the weekend. I guess grandmas just have a special place in Gods big heart!

She was too weak to even remove her shoes. She just mustered enough energy to prop herself in bed and grab the half bottle of whiskey on the table next to the bed. Her Adam's apple bopped up and down as she drained the bottle in a few gulps. She surprised herself when she was able to raise the bottle with a sigh of victory. She picked herself up and head out to the shower. Her mind had shut out the conversation with the doctor. She felt a peace she had not experienced in a long while. Somehow, she felt that she was going to pull through this, for the sake of the four kids and Mark. Just thinking about them feasting on chocolate chip cookies at grannies brought so much joy to her heart.

She turned off the shower and robbed up in red. She then spread the bed afresh and drew the curtains. She put away the empty bottle of whiskey and then slipped into bed. But before she did so, she wrote a silly note for Mark to find when he got home.

"Honey, we didn't bring home a baby, we brought home a cancer!"

Surviving the cancer diagnosis

The next weeks that followed was "life happening to Mary and Mark."

First, relatives who all along had been kept out of the loop had to be brought in. Some were brought in to offer emotional support, others brought in to help with the kids while others just came in for financial support. All the same, the whole extended clan came in!

Second was the chemotherapy itself. Cancer had finally hit home for this close-knit family of six. Despite constant reassurance from the medical team that this was one of the best cancers with great success rates, there was always the fear. When a series of bad things happen to you, you are always primed for the worst. I mean, first, you were among the 0.001% to be a victim of molar pregnancy. Then you became again the 1/68 to have the molar pregnancy develop into cancer. Surely, you might as well be among the percentage that dies from this friendly cancer!

Then you wake up one morning and all you see on your pillow is your precious hair! When you walk into your wardrobe to pick an outfit it takes you a solid thirty minutes as nothing fits! Things you once took for granted such as finishing the food on your plate are now a laudable feat. What's worst is the concoction of drugs that you have been put on that makes you just want to sleep and wake up in 2020 when all this is done and dusted.

Thankfully for Mary, she responded well to the treatment each cycle. Emotionally, she oscillated between being positive and upbeat at the times when she wasn't so beaten down. At other times she just curled up like a ball and hoped for a better day. Her office gave her much support and visited with her regularly. They went as far as organizing a molar pregnancy awareness day at the office in honor of her, where they made cards, did bracelets and planted trees in her honor, how thoughtful!

In no time, everyone at the hospital knew Mary on a first name basis. They had seen her so many times. Unfortunately, the kids drew more and more away. They were like nomads constantly being shuttled from one house to the other to allow their mother enough time to rest and recover in between treatment. The children could see the changes taking place in Mary's body and were very good in sympathizing with her. They took turns in caring for their baby brother and helped in feeding each other. They were best behaved during this time, sensing the tension and pressure that hang heavily on the family. No one dropped the ball. It kind of felt like everyone was trying to bribe God to restore Mary's health and in exchange, everyone would be on their best behavior.

Finding healing

It seems like God heeded to the pleas of the foursome and their dad because six months later, Mary was healed! Also, two years later she still tested negative for tumor markers. She is thriving and so is her family!

A diagnosis of molar pregnancy is frequently received with mixed reactions. They range from a lack of feeling to deep heart-wrenching emotions, and all reactions are perfectly okay. How a person reacts depends on many factors such as prior knowledge on the condition, outlook to life, how far along one had bonded with the pregnancy, how an individual grieves and many other factors.

A molar pregnancy is the beginning of a pregnancy, even if it lacks a viable fetus in it. Therefore, one person justifiably sees it as the loss of an offspring that would have been while another sees it as a pseudopregnancy and therefore not a real pregnancy. These two people may react very differently to the diagnosis of a molar pregnancy, as one is completely torn apart, the other may be strong enough to move on. Still, there is another who thinks that they are not affected at first but later they crumble. These situations make it very difficult even for caregivers to know what kind of support to give to patients of molar pregnancies.

For Mary and Mark, they received the diagnosis with mixed feelings. Thankfully enough for them, they had a good support system that they were able to make good use of before it was too late! They greatly benefitted from the medical staff following up on them and the therapist who they were attached to ended up as a great fit for their needs. As Mary says, they would not have pulled through the cancer diagnosis without the help of the therapist.

That said, other patients have received adequate support from their networks of informed friends and family. Still, others have found great help in reading literature on the topic in the quiet of their closets. All in all, we all react differently to different stressors that we encounter.

Bridging the gap; objectives of the book

This short book aims to bridge the knowledge gap that is characteristic of molar pregnancy.

For the patient of molar pregnancy, this book aims at answering questions about the condition. From scientific questions on the development of molar pregnancy, causes, diagnosis and treatment to emotional questions on grief and coping with the diagnosis.

The aim is to provide a valid resource in terms of a handbook that a patient can turn to after being diagnosed with molar pregnancy. It gives direct answers to questions that the patient may have. It also contains questions that a patient may have but not have found the right words to express. Depending on what stage of the journey the patient is in, some questions may provide foresight as to what lies ahead. These kinds of questions will help the patient in preparing ahead for what is coming.

The questions also probe the hidden emotions of a patient by triggering thoughts and emotions surrounding conception. They explore issue on progression to choriocarcinoma. They also aim at educating a patient on contraception. Importantly, they guide the patient in spotting early signs of depression and how to seek help when the need arises. The book systematically guides the patient through the grieving progress and ensures that they are able to adequately navigate through this phase with positive outcomes.

Lastly, the book prepares that patient for insensitive remarks that may come from caregivers and loved ones.

No one is quite wearing your shoes and hence, no one will quite get it as perfectly as you would wish for them to.

For the partner

When a molar pregnancy happens, two parties are equally as involved, it takes the two to make a baby. Unfortunately, the man is always left out as if he is an ordinary bystander. At most, he is just to be the pillar for the mother to lean on.

This book breaks away from the norm and tries to explore questions that the father may have regarding his own role and place in a molar pregnancy. All questions are complementary to both partners and may help them explore their own and each other's emotions at this critical time. As with the first part, these may be questions a man may be asking himself, some questions he may not have thought of but may be very instrumental in his healing process, now that he has come across the answers.

For caregivers

I have written this book in the capacity of a caregiver, so yes, this book is instrumental for you too as a caregiver. A caregiver may be a medic, social worker, therapist and friends and relatives of molar pregnancy victims. Also, it is important to note that any woman could easily switch from being a caregiver to being a patient in no time. Molar pregnancy can happen to any woman of reproductive age.

The biggest gap between caregivers and patients may not be in the scientific knowledge on molar pregnancy but the emotional impact the condition has on patients and how to address it. It is not enough to have the zeal to help victims walk triumphantly through a molar pregnancy diagnosis, zeal without knowledge is destructive.

A special section of this book is exclusive to questions that a caregiver may have in relation to helping a patient cope with molar pregnancy. However, it is imperative to read the whole book to equip yourself with both the scientific and emotional knowledge on molar pregnancy. By pondering the questions that a patient and her partner may be having regarding the condition you will be better equipped to offer help.

The book also aims to create awareness about molar pregnancy and encourage the discussion about it. When people are better informed about molar pregnancy they will be better placed to ask relevant questions that will spur positive change. Let's talk about molar pregnancy and campaign for better support for affected families.

How the book is formatted

The book is formatted as questions and answers. The questions are slightly more than seventy. The questions are arranged systematically from diagnosis to treatment of molar pregnancy. The questions also include the emotional aspects surrounding molar pregnancy; grief and depression.

The questions are derived from what patients and caregivers have asked on different platforms. Some questions are hypothetical based on knowledge gaps that have been identified. Some questions are deduced from reactions that patients have exhibited after a diagnosis of molar pregnancy.

The book sums up with resourceful links that can give further help for a victim or a caregiver. It also gives guidance on moving on from a molar pregnancy to trying again for another baby, if that is desirable to the couple.

As usual, some questions may not be helpful or applicable to you. You have the right to skip those. Keep what good, discard what you don't "feel with".

Good reading!

22

Chapter Two

WHAT IS MOLAR PREGNANCY?

This section widely explains molar pregnancy from conception to the unfortunate termination of the molar pregnancy. It is formatted as 30 Q&As.

1. Was there a baby in my womb?

The answer to this depends on both subjective and objective factors. The objective factors have to do with the kind of molar pregnancy that was present. For a complete molar pregnancy, only placental tissue is present with no fetal tissue in it. In an incomplete molar pregnancy, there is some fetal tissue present but with gross deformities due to chromosomal abnormalities. As much as the fetal tissue is present and has begun to develop, it is incompatible with life as it lacks maternal chromosomes.

Away with the medical jargon, fetal tissue is either absent or when it is present, it is not viable and therefore cannot develop into a complete child. Pictures of incomplete moles have revealed the formation of teeth and hair and other body parts.

This is the basis of the arguments surrounding molar pregnancies as being or not being real pregnancies. Some argue that life starts at the point of conception whether a baby is formed doesn't matter.

Conclusively, we can say that whatever stance a mother chooses to adopt is legitimate and valid. A mother's or a father's feelings are valid and need to be respected.

So, the answer to the question is, yes there was the beginning of life in your womb, however, it was cut short due to factors beyond your control.

2. What happened to my baby?

The baby in your womb stopped growing at some point, that is, if there was one in the first place, as you may choose to see it.

A complete molar pregnancy occurs when two sperms fertilize an empty egg which is not carrying genetic information. As a result, the pregnancy lacks maternal chromosomes but has double the number of paternal chromosomes. It can develop placental tissues which produce the Hcg hormone. This hormone is responsible for pregnancy symptoms.

For an incomplete molar pregnancy to occur, an egg with faulty chromosomes is fertilized. Therefore, there is the beginning of life as some fetal tissue is formed. However, the placental tissue grows rapidly and overpowers the fetal tissue. On a scan, some fetal parts can be identified.

Molar pregnancies are incompatible with life and most will self-abort at some point. This happens as a spontaneous miscarriage and the product that is expelled will have the appearance of a cluster of grapes.

Because of chromosomal abnormalities, your "baby" did not get a chance to grow either past fertilization or beyond a certain fetal stage. Even when the baby developed past the first trimester, it had significant chromosomal abnormalities that were not compatible with life.

3. Did my baby have a heartbeat?

This again depends on the type of molar pregnancy that you had. In an incomplete mole with fetal parts present, perhaps it did. The heart develops at around day 22 that should be like five weeks after the first day of your last menses. In most cases, the heartbeat will be present until around week nine to ten when a spontaneous abortion normally occurs. At this point, the baby just ceases to grow and must be expelled from the womb. However, in some cases, a molar pregnancy will persist up to four to five months and may require a doctor induced abortion. By this time, there is usually no heartbeat, just the products of conception which mostly comprise of placental tissue that has degenerated into grape-like clusters or cysts.

4. Why is it called a mole?

The term mole is just used to denote the clump of abnormal tissues with a grape like appearance that usually characterizes a molar pregnancy.

The term is not particularly a kind replacement for the fetus or developing baby and it may throw you back when the doctor or nurse uses it, but don't you worry. It is okay to refer to your baby as a baby.

When an ultrasound is performed, your uterus will have an appearance that medically is referred to as a snowstorm appearance. You will be able to visualize clusters of things that appear as grapes. These grapelike vesicles are visible even to the naked eye. When the mass is expelled you will be able to see the grapelike vesicles otherwise referred to as cysts. The grapelike vesicles are formed by the degeneration of the placental tissue.

A molar pregnancy is also referred to as a hydatidiform mole. A hydatid is a fluid-filled cyst. A mole is a cluster of cells. Therefore, a hydatidiform mole is a cluster of fluid-filled cysts.

5. Why was my pregnancy test positive (hcg)?

Pregnancy tests are designed to check for the presence or amount of a pregnancy hormone called human chorionic gonadotropin (hcg). This hormone is produced when a fertilized egg implants on the wall of the uterus. Hcg is only produced in the presence of a pregnancy, whether viable or not.

There are two kinds of pregnancy tests. One tests for just the presence of hcg usually in urine, this is the common strip test and will turn positive from 14 days. The other tests for the exact amount of hcg usually in blood, it is called a beta hcg test.

In the case of a molar pregnancy, since fertilization took place and there was implantation of the fetus, hcg will be produced as usual. The difference is that the hcg will be produced at a much faster rate as the placental tissue is being rapidly generated.

Therefore, a beta hcg test may be able to detect an anomaly that may point towards a molar pregnancy based on the level of hcg present in the blood.

Normally, the amount of hcg should double every two to three days. A higher hcg level than is expected for a particular gestational age may point towards several factors, one of them is a molar pregnancy.

6. Was it my fault or my partner's fault?

It is not very clear as to the real cause of molar pregnancy. Therefore, blame cannot be apportioned.

However, several factors have been identified that may predispose on to having a molar pregnancy.

- Maternal age
- Being below 20 years or over 40 years may predispose you to molar pregnancy.
- Genetic factors
- Chromosomal abnormalities may arise due to various reasons

- Race
- Women from South East Asia, Philippines and Mexico have higher rates of molar pregnancy.
- A previous molar pregnancy
- If you have had a previous molar pregnancy, your chances of getting a subsequent one are slightly higher. However, the likelihood is still minimal.
- Diet
- A diet that lacks adequate amounts of carotene and folic acid may increase your risk for a molar pregnancy.
- White women in the US are at a higher risk of getting a molar pregnancy than black women in the US.
- With this in mind, it would be inappropriate to apportion blame to either of the partners. And thankfully, couples who have had a previous molar pregnancy can still go ahead to have healthy babies after diagnosis and treatment of a molar pregnancy.

7. Why did I feel like I did with my last pregnancy?

Because of the presence of hcg hormone. The symptoms that occur in the first trimester of pregnancy are usually attributable to hcg and other changes as the body adjusts to the pregnancy. Your body may exhibit any of the following symptoms that are similar to those of a normal pregnancy.

- Nausea and vomiting
- Enlarging of the uterus

- Cramping
- Breast changes

You may also get other symptoms that may not be present in a normal pregnancy such as:

- Painful vaginal bleeding
- A larger than expected uterus
- Exaggerated vomiting
- Early preeclampsia
- Symptoms of thyroid disease
- Lack of fetal movements

Other symptoms may be psychological as you are expecting to be pregnant. You may feel fetal movements that may not actually be there. Even after you lose the pregnancy you may still go on to feel like you are pregnant. It is either you have a persistent molar pregnancy which should be treated as a medical emergency or these persisting symptoms could be purely psychological. In case of the latter, you will need to see a therapist or talk to someone about it.

8. Will this happen again?

Chances of recurrence of a molar pregnancy are minimal. That said, the answer is yes! You can get a subsequent molar pregnancy after a first one. Your likelihood of getting a molar pregnancy increases after the first one. Hypothetically, perhaps because you still have the same risk factors that predisposed you the first time around.

Statistically speaking, after a first molar pregnancy, you have a 1.8% chance of getting a subsequent molar pregnancy. In other words, 1 in 55 molar pregnancy patients get a subsequent molar pregnancy. This is a twenty-fold increase down from 0.001% likelihood before any molar pregnancy.

After a second molar pregnancy, you have a 10% chance of getting a third molar pregnancy. Your likelihood increases five times over again.

However, this should not scare you as the chances are still low. Thankfully, you will be followed up after the first molar pregnancy so that signs of recurrence are spotted early, and you can start receiving treatment.

Recurrent molar pregnancies still have good success rates with treatment and you still stand a chance of getting a normal healthy baby after a subsequent molar pregnancy. However, you will need adequate psychological support to get you through this and move on to getting the cherished rainbow baby/babies.

9. Does a molar pregnancy mean that I am infertile?

Absolutely not! In fact, some women have reported that they conceived faster after a molar pregnancy than they had previously. However, this is hypothetical and may not have any scientific backing.

It is important to make it clear that having a molar pregnancy says nothing about your fertility or your partner's. And neither does the diagnosis or treatment of a molar pregnancy affect your fertility.

Even after chemotherapy treatment for an invasive molar pregnancy, it is possible to go ahead to conceive and get a healthy baby.

Molar pregnancies may occur due to chromosomal abnormalities of maternal or paternal genes. The sperm/s may fertilize an empty egg or when the egg has genetic information (not empty) it may still be faulty. When the egg is empty, the paternal chromosomes may duplicate to provide extra chromosomes. This, however, does not imply that all the maternal eggs or paternal sperms are faulty. A couple may still go ahead to have a healthy pregnancy after a previous molar pregnancy.

10. What are D&C and ERPC?

Many times, a molar pregnancy will end up as a spontaneous abortion. This is the body's natural mechanism of expelling the malformed products of conception. This occurs around month four or before but could happen at any time.

When a spontaneous abortion occurs following a pregnancy, you need to report to the hospital for a checkup. Sometimes, some tissue is retained in the uterus after a miscarriage. The doctor will perform a scan to check for any retained tissue. In case there is some tissue retained, it will be removed. ERCP stands for evacuation of retained products on conception. This is the process of removing the retained tissues from the uterus. However, this term is rarely used nowadays as it is not very friendly.

If a molar pregnancy does not miscarry spontaneously, your doctor may give you medication to trigger an abortion. If the abortion fails to happen, he will have to manually remove the pregnancy to avoid any further complications. One of the procedures he may use is vacuum aspiration followed by D&C which stands for dilatation and curettage. This procedure can be done under general or localized anesthesia. The cervix is manually dilated, and the molar pregnancy product is cleaned out. The procedure itself may not be very painful; however, you may opt to get wholly sedated so that you do not have to remain with the memory of the loss. That will be up to you to decide.

11. When will my periods return?

Your periods may return as soon as the molar pregnancy is expelled and your hcg levels return to negative.

However, this may vary with individuals just as the frequency and duration of periods vary from one individual to another.

It is important to understand that your body interpreted the molar pregnancy like a usual pregnancy and will respond in a similar way. In a normal pregnancy, periods return soon after delivery, however, this may be delayed due to breastfeeding which has an antagonistic effect on menses. In a molar pregnancy, the periods should return soon after the expulsion of the molar pregnancy. However, this will only happen if the hcg levels return to a negative level. If the hcg levels persist, the body will go on interpreting this as a pregnancy and you will have no periods.

Other factors such as drugs, stress level, and dietary factors may affect your menses. In case they delay past six months after your hcg levels drop to zero, you should consult your doctor. If they return soon, it means that you are fertile and may need to be started on contraception. The recommended duration for waiting is six months after your hcg levels drop to zero.

12. What if there is a healthy twin or triplets?

In some rare cases, a molar pregnancy may be present together with one or more healthy fetuses. This is due to twinning where one fetus has abnormal placental proliferation while the other twin develops normally.

It is possible for the viable fetus to develop normally and be delivered at term with no obvious physical deformities. Some complications surrounding this pregnancy include bleeding, preterm labor, late abortion, persistent gestational trophoblastic disease and severe anemia in the fetus. The fetus, if it comes to term may also have a low gestational weight for age.

Several factors will determine the viability of the normal fetus. Most importantly is the karyotype or makeup of the chromosomes of the fetus. Other factors include the size of the molar placenta, the rate at which the molar pregnancy is degenerating and circulation in the placenta. Sometimes fetal circulation from the viable twin is sufficient but becomes compromised in the last trimester as the size of the fetus increases.

That said, it is possible to have a healthy and viable twin that grows to term. If this is diagnosed early, a mother should be closely monitored for any complications that may arise.

13. What complications should I expect?

After the removal of a molar pregnancy either spontaneously or induced, the hcg levels should drop to zero. If this fails to happen, it could be indicative of a persistent gestational trophoblastic disease.

This happens when the uterus goes on to produce hcg even after the expulsion of a molar pregnancy. The uterus may go on to produce abnormal tissues.

In some cases, (invasive mole) the molar pregnancy burrows deep into the uterine wall and part of the tissues may remain even after D&C. In these cases, there may be hemorrhage into the abdominal cavity and a pelvic exam needs to be performed to rule this out. These remaining tissues may be responsible for the persistent hcg levels and can be treated with chemotherapy. If treatment for persistent GTD is initiated early, success rates are almost at 100%.

In some rare instances (2-3% of cases), the persistent molar pregnancy turns out to be cancerous. When the cancer is confined to the uterus, chemotherapy treatment is very effective, and you may still retain childbearing capabilities. If cancer has spread to other organs, chemotherapy treatment may still be effective with a 75%-85% chance of remission. But fertility may be compromised, and a removal of the uterus may be necessary.

Methotrexate is the commonly used drug for chemotherapy.

14. How will the doctor tell if it is a molar pregnancy?

Unfortunately, most times a molar pregnancy is diagnosed after what appeared to be a normal miscarriage. That is why it is important to have follow-up care after a miscarriage to avoid any complications associated with a molar pregnancy. And even when there are no after complications, it is good to have it for the record, because the risk for a second molar pregnancy increases after a first molar pregnancy. Not that this information is of encouragement to you, but may be helpful to know.

If the molar pregnancy is discovered before a miscarriage happens, a pelvic scan will reveal the following.

Complete mole

- Lacking fetal parts
- Lacking amniotic fluid
- Grapelike appearance of the placenta almost filling the uterus
- Possible cysts in the ovaries
- No heartbeat at all

Incomplete mole

- Fetal parts may be present

- Low levels of amniotic fluid
- Grapelike appearance of the uterus
- No heartbeat past nine weeks

The doctor may also ask for samples of your blood to measure hcg levels. They should be abnormally high in a molar pregnancy.

The doctor may also interview you for other symptoms that could be indicative of a molar pregnancy.

15. For how long will my Hcg levels be monitored?

The aim of closely monitoring hcg levels is to confirm the success of treatment for molar pregnancy and identify early signs of persistent gestational trophoblastic disease. Other than monitoring of beta hcg levels, a pelvic ultrasound may also be routinely performed to rule out persistent GTD.

Incomplete molar pregnancies have a residual chance of persisting after a uterine evacuation (1.2-4%). Metastasis is even less frequent.

Complete molar pregnancies have a higher chance of developing into a persistent GTD after a uterine evacuation.

The risk of persistent GTD is usually high in the first twelve months following a molar pregnancy, most cases will present before six months.

While hcg levels are being monitored, it is important that you be on contraception. Most forms of contraception other than an intra-uterine device should be acceptable to use. If you get pregnant during this period when your hcg levels are still being monitored, it may take longer to spot signs of persistent GTD. A subsequent pregnancy will also produce hcg and it may be hard to tell the difference between the two. In case this happens, ultrasonography can be used to identify the presence of another pregnancy.

Ideally, your hcg levels should be monitored for an additional six months from when the levels drop to zero. If they do not increase within this period, you will be given a clean bill of health to move on.

16. What if I get pregnant before six months?

It could be okay, as long as your hcg levels had fallen to zero. But you will have to cross your fingers that there was no invasive mole or persistent GTD that had not been detected. In the unfortunate event that there was, this could seriously complicate your following pregnancy.

On the positive side where there was no persistent GTD, you will need to inform your doctor. You will then be closely monitored to ensure that there is no recurrence of a molar pregnancy. By week six, the doctor can rule out a complete molar pregnancy if there is a heartbeat. By week ten, some genetic tests can be performed to rule out an incomplete mole. Your pregnancy should then proceed as normal.

On the negative side, if you have persistent GTD, you may get a subsequent molar pregnancy and have to go through the same treatment process as before. Then you will have chemotherapy after that. It is unlikely that you have a normal pregnancy coexisting with a persistent GTD.

The good news is, you can still have a healthy baby after your treatment is complete.

17. What contraception should I use before six months?

It is controversial whether the hormones in the contraceptive pill accelerate the growth of trophoblastic tissue. For this reason, you should avoid contraceptive pills and other hormonal methods until your hcg levels have stabilized at negative levels. This also applies to patients on chemotherapy for persistent GTD treatment. If you happen to conceive while you are receiving chemotherapy, your baby will have a higher risk for fetal/teratogenic deformities. In simpler terms, the chemotherapy drugs can cross the placental barrier and affect the normal formation of your baby.

IUCDs may also not be recommended as the uterus may need adequate time to heal.

Barrier methods and spermicides are completely safe to use. In case you do not desire to have another child, a complete hysterectomy (removal of the uterus) may be ideal for you. This will not only serve as a permanent birth control method, it will also decrease your likelihood of developing persistent GTD or choriocarcinoma.

Ultimately, you should consult your doctor on an appropriate contraception method for you. The use of hormonal methods is controversial as some studies have proven that it is indeed safe to use them during follow-up for molar pregnancy.

18. Which danger signs should you look out for during follow up?

The diagnosis of a molar pregnancy is usually a big scare, not just because of the loss of a pregnancy but also because of the associated cancer risk.

As your hcg levels are being monitored, you need to be on the lookout for the following signs that may point towards a persistent GTD.

For recurrent complete molar pregnancy

- Vaginal bleeding
- Anemia
- Nausea and vomiting
- Distended uterus
- Signs of a hyperactive thyroid

For recurrent incomplete molar pregnancy

- Nausea and vomiting
- Vaginal bleeding
- Anemia
- Swelling of the abdomen

For invasive moles and choriocarcinoma

- Vaginal bleeding

- Bleeding into the abdominal cavity which can only be seen with a scan
- Anemia
- Signs of infection
- Abdominal swelling
- Lung symptoms such as chest pain, dry cough, difficulty in breathing. This is in the presence of metastasis to the lung.
- Presence of a vaginal mass in case of spread to the vagina
- Another like site of metastasis is the brain. In this case, you will have symptoms such as persistent headaches, projectile vomiting, dizziness, seizures etc.

Make sure you inform your doctor of any symptoms you may observe during your follow up. The earlier the signs of a persistent GTD are detected, the better the outcomes of treatment.

19. What is a complete mole?

A molar pregnancy could either be complete or partial. A complete molar pregnancy may be referred to as a diploid molar pregnancy while an incomplete molar pregnancy is referred to as a triploid molar pregnancy. This is because of the sets of chromosomes present in each case.

There are two probabilities that would cause a complete molar pregnancy to occur. In 90% of the cases, a single sperm fertilizes an egg that has lost its genetic or chromosomal information. The sperm will then duplicate itself to produce an extra set of chromosomes. In 10% of cases, two sperms will fertilize an egg that has lost its genetic or chromosomal information. In both cases, the fetus will lack maternal chromosomes and have the following characteristics.

Complete mole

- Lacking fetal parts
- Lacking amniotic fluid
- Grapelike appearance of the placenta almost filling the uterus
- Possible cysts in the ovaries
- No heartbeat at all
- Signs of hyperthyroidism
- Signs of pre-eclampsia

By week six, it is possible to confirm the diagnosis of a complete molar pregnancy by an ultrasound. An ultrasound will reveal a snow storm/ cluster grape appearance. Also, there will be no fetal heartbeat present. A complete molar pregnancy has a higher chance of developing into a persistent GTD and choriocarcinoma.

20. What is a partial mole?

For a partial molar pregnancy to occur, two sperms or one sperm that reduplicates itself fertilizes a haploid egg. As a result, the resulting embryo has an excess of chromosomes. Due to this genetic anomaly, the embryo will have deformities that are not compatible with life. Just like a complete molar pregnancy, a partial molar pregnancy is not viable. It will present with the following signs:

- Fetal parts may be present
- Low levels of amniotic fluid
- Grapelike appearance of the uterus
- No heartbeat past nine weeks

It is important to note that both complete and partial molar pregnancies will present with other pregnancy-related symptoms such as nausea and vomiting, enlarged uterus, missed periods, increase in weight and positive testing for pregnancy.

Partial molar pregnancy has a lower chance of developing into a persistent GTD as compared to a complete molar pregnancy.

21. What is an invasive mole?

Sometimes, a molar pregnancy burrows deep into the cervical tissue. When this happens, it is referred to as an invasive mole. An invasive mole is also considered to be a tumor that has not yet metastasized to other regions. However, it is still a neoplasm and can spread to other organs and so it needs to be treated as a medical emergency when identified.

Diagnosis of an invasive mole may be made after a molar pregnancy has been previously diagnosed. It is a complication of both complete and partial molar pregnancies, but with a higher occurrence following a complete molar pregnancy. Beta hcg levels will keep increasing even after expulsion of the molar pregnancy. Other symptoms that may be indicative of an invasive mole include:

- Bleeding into the abdominal cavity which may appear with ultrasonography
- Persistent nausea and vomiting
- Anemia
- Vaginal bleeding
- Severe pain in the abdomen

Treatment for an invasive mole is by chemotherapy. Methotrexate is the commonly used drug. Depending on how much of the uterus has been invaded, your doctor may deem it necessary to perform a hysterectomy to remove the uterus completely.

Success rates for treatment are almost at 100% for non-complicated cases. It is still possible to conceive and deliver a healthy baby after diagnosis and treatment for an invasive mole.

21. How soon can I try for another baby?

As soon as your doctor gives you a clean bill of health to try again. This will be after he has monitored your hcg levels for a period that is satisfactory to him/her.

It is important to note that having a molar pregnancy does not in any way interfere with your fertility. You may be able to conceive soon after diagnosis and treatment for a molar pregnancy.

However, conceiving before the required time may pose serious threats your health and that of your baby. First, you are at a higher risk of developing a subsequent molar pregnancy. This should not scare you as the chance is still 1 in 55 cases. Because of this, your subsequent pregnancies will be high risk and will be closely monitoring.

Secondly, a subsequent pregnancy is going to cause your hcg levels to rise again. This will make it very difficult for your doctor to differentiate between a persistent gestational trophoblastic disease and subsequent pregnancy.

Thirdly, in case you conceive while receiving treatment for persistent GTD, your baby will be at risk of developing serious deformities. Chemotherapy drugs have been established to cause teratogenic effects.

Lastly, your body requires adequate time to heal and readjust to a healthy state after the diagnosis and treatment of molar pregnancy. It is therefore advisable that you use contraception until the doctor is satisfied that you are safe to try again for another baby.

Not all hope is lost in case you conceive before you have been given a clean bill of health. Many women have been there and were able to get healthy babies, remember the odds of recurrence are not against you, it is still 1 in 55 women that get a recurrence.

22. Is a molar pregnancy a tumor?

Yes, it is a benign tumor that can develop into cancer, but the likelihood is minimal.

A tumor is basically a mass of rapidly diving cells while a mole is a cluster of abnormal placental tissues. That said, a benign tumor is not cancerous unless it develops metastatic capabilities. This means that as much as a mole can be referred to as a tumor, in most cases it is benign. It is only in a small percentage of cases that a molar pregnancy becomes cancerous.

Because of the likelihood that it can develop into cancer, a molar pregnancy will be closely monitored until all chances of developing into a cancer are ruled out. Molar pregnancies account for 50% of choriocarcinomas. Complete molar pregnancies and subsequent molar pregnancies will increase your risk of developing choriocarcinoma.

If you have a molar pregnancy and it, unfortunately, ends up becoming cancer, you need not worry. Choriocarcinoma is highly treatable with chemotherapy and in rare circumstances, it may be combined with radiation therapy. As long as you comply with follow up care after molar pregnancy treatment, your doctor should be able to detect early cancer signs and start you on treatment.

The good news is that you should still be able to conceive and deliver a normal baby even after treatment for choriocarcinoma.

23. How does a miscarriage happen?

Both complete and partial molar pregnancies are not viable pregnancies. The molar pregnancy due to chromosomal abnormalities cannot develop into a normal baby. In fact, most complete molar pregnancies will not form any fetal tissues. A partial molar pregnancy may form fetal tissue and even have a heartbeat which will be lost at around week ten.

In some instances, the molar pregnancy may continue to grow undetected as a mole until month four or five. In other instances, it will be expelled soon after week nine or ten.

A miscarriage is the process by which a pregnancy is involuntarily expelled from a mother's body. The medical term for a miscarriage is a spontaneous abortion. Most molar pregnancies end up as miscarriages. You will know you are having a miscarriage if:

- You experience vaginal spotting which may have a red to brownish color
- You have abdominal cramps
- You have lower back pain
- You expel clots from the vagina
- You feel light headed
- You may have severe vaginal bleeding

Some factors that may increase your risk of a miscarriage are:

- Chromosomal abnormalities such as in molar pregnancy
- Incompetent cervix
- Polycystic ovary syndrome
- Underlying health conditions

When the body senses that the pregnancy is not viable, it may trigger a miscarriage to expel the pregnancy. In case a molar pregnancy does not miscarry naturally, once it is discovered the doctor will give you a pill to induce an abortion. This will be followed by a D&C to clean the uterus of all remains of the molar pregnancy.

24. If I miscarried in the past, could it have been an undiagnosed molar Pregnancy?

Yes, it can, that is why it is important to have a follow up after a miscarriage.

Having a miscarriage can be quite devastating. But what could be more devastating is discovering that the miscarriage was a molar pregnancy. It is normal for this to throw you into panic mode, not only must you wait for six months to a year before you can try again, but you also stand a higher chance of a recurrent molar pregnancy. More to this, you also have a higher risk of developing choriocarcinoma.

Thankfully, doctors will routinely follow up on all patients after a miscarriage and will able to detect if it the miscarriage was a normal pregnancy. In case it is discovered to be a molar pregnancy, you will be informed and thereafter you will be closely monitored for the development of persistent GTD.

If you suspect that a previous miscarriage could have been a molar pregnancy that was not diagnosed, you need not worry. If you developed no further symptoms and it has been a while since the miscarriage, chances are you did not develop a persistent GTD. Symptoms of a persistent GTD tend to show within a year after the expulsion of a molar pregnancy. More accurately, symptoms should appear within six months.

In case six months have not elapsed since your miscarriage and you are not on follow up, it is advisable to consult your doctor and he may advise to have your hcg levels checked.

25. Could I have done anything to save this baby?

Not really. Both types of molar pregnancies have little to no viability potential. In a complete molar pregnancy, the fetus lacks any maternal chromosomes. The paternal chromosomes may duplicate to give an extra set of chromosomes. The paternal chromosomes will only give rise to placental tissues that will proliferate at a fast rate and later degenerate to form fluid-filled vesicles that have a grape like appearance. In most cases, no fetal parts or amniotic fluid is present.

In a partial molar pregnancy, a haploid egg is fertilized by one or two sperms. As a result, the fetus has three sets of chromosomes (triploid). This overload of genetic information will cause the fetus to have abnormalities that are not compatible with life. Fetal parts will develop but will be overshadowed by placental tissues. The fetus may develop a heartbeat which may be present until week ten.

Because of these chromosomal deformities, there is nothing you can do to "save this baby". It is just not a viable pregnancy.

However, in some cases of partial molar pregnancies, a viable fetus may exist together with the incomplete mole. In this case, it is possible for the viable fetus to grow and be delivered as a healthy baby, but you be closely monitored.

26. Should I change my nutrition?

A diet that lacks folate and carotene is one of the risk factors for molar pregnancy.

Carotene is a form of vitamin A. It is essential for the growth and differentiation of many cells and tissues. Oranges and dark green vegetables are good sources of carotene.

Folate is the synthetic form of vitamin B9. It plays a big role in preventing neural tube defects or severe defects of the brain and spinal cord. Every pregnant woman needs to take folate pre-conceptions. It may also lower your baby's risk for other birth defects such as cleft lip and palate. Finally, it plays a significant role in the formation and repair of DNA. This is the genetic makeup of the cell and could be the source of the relationship with molar pregnancy.

It may be difficult to pinpoint the greatest risk factor that may have predisposed you to molar pregnancy. That said, seeing the potential benefits of beta-carotene and folate, there is no harm in incorporating them into your diet, especially if you are trying again for another baby. Foods rich in folate include chickpeas, liver, lentils, spinach, asparagus, avocado and beets. In case your diet is already rich in folate and carotene, it's okay. Diet is just one of the risk factors for a molar pregnancy. Other factors could be way beyond your control.

27. Is my daughter more predisposed to molar pregnancy if I had one?

Heredity is not really a risk factor for molar pregnancies, the association is farfetched. Known risk factors for molar pregnancy include:

- Maternal age; being below 20 and above 35 increases your risk for molar pregnancy.
- Chromosomal abnormalities
- A diet low in folate and carotene increases your risk for molar pregnancy.
- A previous molar pregnancy will increase your chances for a subsequent molar pregnancy.
- Race and geographic location.
- White women in the US have a higher chance of developing molar pregnancy.
- Women from Southeast Asia have eight times higher chance of getting a molar pregnancy.
- Women from Mexico and the Philippines have a higher chance of getting a molar pregnancy than women from the US.

Your daughter may have a similar chance as you of developing a molar pregnancy, because she may be within the same geographical location, eat a similar diet, be of similar weight etc. but not solely because of genetic or heredity factors.

28. How come no one ever mentioned this to me before?

Unfortunately, there is little awareness regarding molar pregnancy. Several factors could contribute to this.

First is the low incidence as compared to other conditions. Not much has been researched or published about molar pregnancies. It is not until recently that aggressive measures were instituted to collect molar pregnancy data and publish it.

Secondly, without adequate follow up care, it may be hard to track all molar pregnancy cases and document them. This is especially true in developing nations where many molar pregnancy cases are unaccounted for.

Lastly, there is the painful assumption that since molar pregnancies are not viable in the first place, the loss isn't a real loss. As a result, victims are not encouraged to talk about their experiences and loss. This is very unfair as the loss may be even more painful as it is complicated by a possibility of a cancer diagnosis.

The silence needs to be broken and more awareness created about molar pregnancy. Awareness can be created by victims, their partners, and caregivers. Every pregnant woman needs to be informed about the risks of molar pregnancy and what signs and symptoms to be on the lookout for.

29. What next after this?

Trying for a rainbow baby if that is your desire!

If you have successfully gone through diagnosis, treatment and follow up care after a molar pregnancy, and have finally been given a clean bill of health, kudos to you! It is not an easy journey and you deserve a pat on the back for pulling through. Have no fear, you are not alone in this. Many women have walked this path and emerged victorious. In case your journey took you through a cancer scare or actual cancer, followed by chemotherapy with all its associated baggage, then yours is even a bigger crown. Not many would have weathered through this and come out alive! But you have.

You need to get out there and share your story that will encourage another woman on this journey.

You need to get out there and write your story that will create awareness and educate somebody who will be a caregiver to a patient tomorrow.

If you are up to trying for your rainbow baby, why not. Some women have conceived faster after a molar pregnancy than before. You may be one of them, keep trying!

Let your success story begin today. Turn your pain into joy by looking at this event from a different angle, that you survived to tell the story and be of encouragement to another woman out there. Isn't that what life is all about?

Lastly, be grateful for the gift of life, now that you understand that indeed it is a gift. So much goes into the creation of life, nothing just happens. So be grateful for who you are and what you have today. Life indeed is one rare privilege, and so is motherhood!

References

Web MD – What is molar pregnancy?

Mayo clinic – Molar pregnancy symptoms and causes

American pregnancy – Molar pregnancy

Cancer research UK – About molar pregnancy

NCBI – Management of molar pregnancy

Chapter three

Invasive mole AND CHORIOCARCINOMA

Perhaps the most devastating thing after the loss of a molar pregnancy is the looming uncertainty of a cancer diagnosis. As if it is not enough to have lost a pregnancy, you still must deal with the possibility of cancer and the subsequent intensive treatment regimen. This could also cause you to despair of ever having a normal pregnancy afterward.

All hope is not lost. If an invasive mole or choriocarcinoma is detected early enough, cure is possible. You can then go on to conceive and deliver a healthy baby after it's all done and dusted. It is important that you are aware of the symptoms and signs that point towards either of these conditions, so you can be started on treatment early enough.

If there is any such a thing as favorite cancer, choriocarcinoma should be it.

Even in the unfortunate event where the choriocarcinoma has metastasized to vital organs, cure is still possible.

This section explores 14 questions surrounding the diagnosis, treatment and follow-up care for invasive mole and choriocarcinoma. It also gives tips for finding hope and reassurance following this heart-breaking diagnosis.

30. Is invasive mole same as choriocarcinoma?

No, the two are different but related as they are both complications of molar pregnancy.

Sometimes a molar pregnancy burrows deep into the uterine tissues. This is what is called an invasive mole. It is a form of persistent gestational trophoblastic disease. Even after treatment of the molar pregnancy, these molar cells remain in the uterus and continues to produce hcg. The persistent molar cells could cause further complications if left untreated. Diagnosis is made by monitoring hcg levels after treatment for a molar pregnancy. If hcg levels fail to drop after the termination of a molar pregnancy, it could point towards an invasive mole.

However, invasive mole should not be confused with retained molar pregnancy after curettage. If a part of the molar pregnancy is not evacuated from the uterus, it will go on to produce hcg and cause other symptoms such as bleeding. But this may not require chemotherapy treatment as the cells are not burrowed deep in the uterine tissues. Invasive moles are more common after a complete molar pregnancy than after a partial molar pregnancy. If an invasive mole is not treated it can become a choriocarcinoma.

A choriocarcinoma, on the other hand, occurs when the molar tissue persists after treatment and becomes cancerous. A choriocarcinoma can spread to other vital organs such as the brain, lungs or liver. Diagnosis is made by monitoring hcg levels after a molar pregnancy and performing a tissue biopsy. Like invasive moles, choriocarcinomas have a higher incidence following a complete molar pregnancy.

Both invasive moles and choriocarcinomas are treated with chemotherapy. They both have a good response rate to treatment, especially if the treatment is initiated early enough.

31. How likely am I to get choriocarcinoma?

Choriocarcinomas are a type of gestational trophoblastic disease.

50% of choriocarcinomas occur following a molar pregnancy.

If you had a complete molar pregnancy, you have an increased chance of getting choriocarcinoma than if you had a partial molar pregnancy.

Choriocarcinomas grow quite fast. They occur in the uterus and will spread to other organs such as the brain, liver, and lungs.

The following symptoms will make you suspect a choriocarcinoma:

- Increasing hcg levels even after the expulsion of molar pregnancy
- Vaginal bleeding

- Foul smelling vaginal discharge
- Abdominal swelling
- Vaginal mass
- Respiratory symptoms
- Coughing up blood
- Chest pain

If you develop any of these symptoms after a molar pregnancy, you need to inform your doctor who will perform further tests.

Several factors, not just molar pregnancy, could increase your risk for choriocarcinoma. The other factors include:

- Molar pregnancy accounts for 50% of cases
- Having a spontaneous abortion accounts for 20%
- Having an ectopic pregnancy accounts for 2%
- A normal pregnancy

After a molar pregnancy, you need to be on follow up for at least six to twelve months to rule out the possibility of a choriocarcinoma. Fortunately, when diagnosed early, cure rates are almost 100%.

32. What is the treatment for invasive mole?

An invasive mole occurs when a molar pregnancy burrows into the uterine tissues. Diagnosis is usually made when hcg levels fail to drop to negative levels after treatment for molar pregnancy. This will be followed by more definitive tests such an ultrasound, CT, MRI or tissue biopsy.

The treatment for an invasive mole needs to be commenced as soon as the diagnosis is made to prevent it from developing further into a choriocarcinoma.

Chemotherapy is the usual treatment for invasive mole. Most commonly used chemotherapy drug is methotrexate which is given until hcg levels drop to negative levels.

The other treatment you will need is symptom controls

Pain relievers such as opioids may be prescribed for pain control. Drugs to control nausea and vomiting may also be prescribed.

Sometimes the invasive mole burrows through the walls of the uterus and causes abdominal bleeding. You will require an abdominal scan to confirm this. You may require surgery to fix this and you will also be put on iron and folate in case your blood loss is significant.

Throughout this process, it is important not to overlook your psychological wellbeing. Be on the lookout for symptoms of depression and alert your therapist consistently on how you are doing emotionally and psychologically. This could be wearing down on you without your knowledge and if not addressed, it could lead to depression.

33. What treatment options are available for choriocarcinoma?

About fifty years ago, choriocarcinoma had a 95% mortality rate. Currently, the cure rate is at 90-95%! Similar to the treatment for an invasive mole, chemotherapy is used.

When choriocarcinoma is confined to the uterus, methotrexate is used as the drug of choice. It is given until hcg levels return to negative levels.

If the cancer has spread from the uterus to other organs, methotrexate will be combined with other drugs to increase efficiency. Depending on how the cancer is staged, total removal of the uterus may be necessary before chemotherapy is commenced.

When metastasis is present in organs such as the brain, radiation therapy may first be performed on these organs. Therefore, in severe cases, a combination of surgery, chemotherapy and radiation therapy may be used. However, this happens in very rare circumstances, and mostly when the diagnosis was made when it was too late.

Choriocarcinoma is a first spreading cancer but it is highly treatable if treatment is initiated early enough. The issue of timing cannot be overemphasized.

Just as with invasive mole treatment, you will be put on other drugs to control your symptoms such as opioids for pain control.

You will also need plenty of psychological support throughout this journey. Dealing with the diagnosis of a molar pregnancy, then cancer, then possibly losing your fertility during treatment cannot be taken lightly. Therefore, it is advisable to have a good support network that may include a personal therapist.

34. What does chemotherapy feel like?

It can be very devastating to have a cancer diagnosis after the diagnosis of a molar pregnancy. You will need a lot of support to get through this. The good news is that others have gotten through it successfully and so can you.

Chemotherapy will have an impact on your physical, emotional, psychological, sexual and even economic well-being.

- Physical symptoms related to use of methotrexate will include hair loss, nausea, and vomiting, loss of appetite, loss of weight, changes in the texture of your skin, mouth sores and diarrhea. The good news is that these side effects will go away as soon as the drug is discontinued.
- Sexual symptoms related to the disease process and treatment will present as diminished sexual appetite.
- Emotionally you may have mood swings depending on the impact of the chemotherapy drugs. This may be characterized by frequent meltdowns after a period of "being okay".
- Psychological symptoms may include the inability to focus and increased stress levels
- Economically, you may not have the energy to go to work while receiving treatment. Treatment will also involve frequent admissions that may disrupt your work.

That said, it is nothing that you can't get through and fortunately treatment does not take a long time if you respond well to the drugs.

35. Can I conceive a healthy baby after chemotherapy?

Yes, you can!

In the unlikely event that you conceive while on chemotherapy, it could pose a serious problem. Chemotherapy drugs can cross the placental barrier and cause teratogenic effects on the developing baby. The baby can become seriously malformed.

If you conceive after successfully completing chemotherapy, you should be safe. In 90-95% of cases, the choriocarcinoma is successfully treated and your body goes back to functioning normally. You should expect your periods to return to normal as soon as hcg levels are below negative and you can try again for your rainbow baby.

It is only in the unfortunate event where you had to have a complete hysterectomy (you had your uterus removed) that your fertility will be affected as you will not be able to carry a normal pregnancy for yourself. But even here, you can consider having a surrogate to "loan you a womb".

However, you still stand a 10% chance of developing a subsequent molar pregnancy. This should not worry you. It only means that after you conceive, you will need to be followed up closely so that signs of a molar pregnancy will be detected early. Remember that the chance is still low.

It is advisable to join support groups of mothers trying to conceive after chemotherapy for molar pregnancy. Such groups are available on Facebook, WhatsApp and baby center.

36. How can I effectively prepare for chemotherapy?

Chemotherapy is an intense process both physically and psychologically. Physically, the drugs used to destroy cancer cells will definitely have side effects that will wear you down and cause bodily changes. You may also find that you are not feeding well as your appetite is diminished. This will make you weak and not able to do many things for yourself. Because of this, you need to prepare in advance before commencing chemotherapy treatment.

Here are a few tips to guide you:

- Before treatment, make sure your body is in good shape. Feed adequately and get as much rest as you can.
- Your doctor may prescribe iron and folate to boost your blood levels as chemotherapy may cause you to have anemia.
- Make sure you see your dentist to rule out any signs of infection. Being on chemotherapy will lower your immunity and cause existing infections to flare up.
- Undergo tests and procedures to make sure that your body is fit enough to handle chemotherapy. Better outcomes are achieved in healthier patients than with sickly patients.
- Plan ahead for side effects.
- Delegate responsibilities at home and at work. Have someone take over your daily responsibilities so that you will not be under pressure once on treatment.

37. I'm I more likely to get other cancers?

Yes and no.

Having choriocarcinoma will not increase your risk for other cancers. But cancer may spread from the womb to affect other vital organs

Likely areas for metastasis of choriocarcinoma are:

- The brain
- When choriocarcinoma spreads to the brain it will present with symptoms such as severe headaches, feeling of lightheadedness, projectile vomiting, fits and blurred vision.
- Treatment will include radiation therapy to the affected part of the brain. This may be combined with surgery and chemotherapy.
- The lungs
- When choriocarcinoma spreads to the lungs, it will present with the following symptoms: difficulty in breathing, chest pain, and persistent dry cough.
- Other regions that a choriocarcinoma could spread to include the vagina and the liver.

Thankfully, even when choriocarcinoma has metastasized to other regions, it is still treatable. Once you have been treated for choriocarcinoma you will remain on follow up to ensure that cancer remains in remission. Beta hcg is the tumor marker for choriocarcinoma and the levels will be monitored perhaps over a couple of years. Cure rates for choriocarcinoma when treatment is initiated early is 90-95%.

38. Is cancer painful?

Yes, most forms of cancer can cause severe pain. Choriocarcinoma is no exception, especially when it has spread to other organs.

Cancer pain could arise due to the tumor pressing onto nerves.

Fortunately, even the most severe forms of cancer pain can be controlled with a good pain control strategy. When devising a plan for pain control, it is important to consider the emotional component of cancer pain.

Mild pain can be adequately controlled using paracetamol or an NSAID.

Moderate pain can be controlled using tramadol.

Severe pain can be controlled using opioids such as Demerol or fentanyl.

The pain drugs could also be combined for better results. It is important to understand the quality of the pain as well as the degree of severity. Bone pain, for example, will present as a sharp burning pain and may indicate that the cancer has spread to the bones.

Pain control should also be accompanied by psychological support. The psychological impact of cancer is so severe that it may sometimes present as actual physical pain. This is also because many patients anticipate severe pain after a cancer diagnosis.

Not all cancers present with pain. If pain is present, it can be sufficiently controlled. Do not hesitate to talk to your physician/oncologist about pain that is not adequately controlled.

39. How will the doctor tell if I am cured?

After chemotherapy, the doctor will go on to monitor your beta hcg levels, the tumor maker for choriocarcinoma. In case you show no improvement in hcg levels after the first cycle of chemotherapy with methotrexate, you may be put on a second cycle and so forth. Also, your oncologist may opt to use a combination of chemotherapy drugs. Your body needs to be in good physical shape each time before each cycle is commenced.

Your doctor will also need to confirm that the cancer had not spread to other organs. He can do this by performing tissue biopsies and checking for signs and symptoms of metastasis.

It is important here to dispel the myth that cancers are incurable. On the contrary, many cancers are curable if detected early enough. Unfortunately, cancers don't show any signs initially, they only begin to exhibit symptoms when the cancer cells have been proliferating long enough in the body to create a mass. The more advanced the cancer is, the harder it is to cure. Also, different types of cancers spread at different rates. Some cancers are fast spreading while others are slow.

Choriocarcinoma is one of the less vicious types of cancer. It has been hypothesized that this is because the cells of cancer only contain paternal chromosomes and so are easy to destroy using chemotherapy.

40. Does my genetic makeup increase my risk for choriocarcinoma?

50% of choriocarcinomas are attributable to molar pregnancies. The rest arise due to various other risk factors.

It is hard to establish the specific cause of many cancers. What exists are risk factors that may predispose you to a specific cancer.

For choriocarcinoma, the following risk factors may predispose you:

If you have a molar pregnancy and have a positive history of cancer in your family, do not fret. With the low incidence of the disease, the odds are still favorable for you.

41. What dietary changes should I make?

As discussed above, lack of adequate amounts of carotene and folate can increase your likelihood of a molar pregnancy and consequently choriocarcinoma.

Other food compounds have also demonstrated the ability to prevent cancer or slow down the spread of choriocarcinoma. They include leafy green vegetables, cruciferous vegetables, berries, squash, sweet potatoes, mushrooms, wheatgrass, nuts and seeds and fresh herbs and spices.

When receiving treatment for invasive mole or choriocarcinoma, the state of your body physically plays a big role. If your body is too weak, your outcome for cancer treatment may be less favorable. A healthy body will give a better prognosis for cancer treatment.

Being deliberate about nutrition will go a long way in preparing you for chemo and in the healing process following chemotherapy and other cancer treatments.

42. What lifestyle changes should I make?

Now that you have lived through and survived invasive mole and choriocarcinoma, life has just begun for you!

You need to be more positive towards life and whatever it brings your way because unlike many people, you have lived through a near-death experience.

You need to be more health conscious. Be careful about what you eat, because we are what we eat. Exercise and maintain your body in the best shape possible.

You also need to have regular cancer screening to rule out the possibility of a recurrence.

43. What if my cancer is not curable?

All hope is not lost in this highly unlikely event.

If your cancer specialist informs you that your cancer is too far spread, do not despair. Palliative care can offer you comfort even as you face the difficult diagnosis.

Palliative care is the care given to patients to improve their quality of life and enrich their experience of life even when an option for a cure is not forthcoming.

It entails relieving the physical symptoms by using medicines. It also involves giving emotional and psychological support to the patient and close family.

Lastly, it prepares the patient to face the reality of death and plan for it.

Ask your doctor to refer you to a good palliative care program near you.

References

American Cancer Society - What is gestational trophoblastic disease?

Cancer Research UK- About gestational Trophoblastic Disease

National Cancer Institute- Gestational Trophoblastic disease Treatment

ASCO- Gestational Trophoblastic Disease: Symptoms and signs

Medline Plus – Tumors and Pregnancy

Foundation for women's cancer - GTD

Chapter four

DEALING WITH GRIEF, LOSS, AND DEPRESSION

For most women, the announcement of a pregnancy comes with a lot of hope and enthusiasm at the prospects of being a mom, or a mom again! Whether planned for or not planned for, a woman's heart warms up to the baby she is carrying in her womb as this is one rare privilege. A woman gets to participate in the creation of life! She begins to change how she walks and dresses and begins to make long-term plans for the arrival of this bundle of joy. Nothing can quite compare to this feeling.

Therefore, when you are told, "Ma' I'm sorry, there is no baby in your womb" the news may just refuse to sink in. I remember one woman insisting that she could still hear her baby kicking in her womb!

Whatever way you receive the news of a molar pregnancy, it always throws you off because no one expects to be in this 0.001%, right? But it did happen to you, and now you have to find a way to cope and move on.

It should be clear that whether you are the kind that breaks down or the kind that takes it in stride and quickly moves on, it is important to seek psychological counseling. This is because grief likes to hide and when it comes out after being concealed for a long time, it is ugly! Some people will grieve for a long time while others will grieve for a very short time. This is perfectly in order.

This section contains 20 real questions, sentiments, feeling and a representation of the emotions that a parent goes through after the diagnosis of a molar pregnancy. It is aimed at exploring all these mixed feelings that you may have expressed or even some that you do not know exist. It may be beneficial to discuss this section with a qualified therapist or a close confidant who can help you realize your own emotions in these matters. Sometimes healing comes through asking questions and finding answers within ourselves.

Whether you chose to see a therapist or not, and whether you feel you need to grieve or not, it is vital to explore your own emotions for you to find healing.

44. What are grief and mourning?

Grief is the strong and overwhelming emotion that most people experience after experiencing a significant loss. The loss could be the death of a significant person in their lives. It could also be the loss of a job, a pet, a home, a marriage, a significant relationship etc. It could also occur after a terminal diagnosis or other significantly devastating news.

Mourning is how people express their grief. How people mourn varies from one person to another. As some will openly display their grief, other will try to conceal it.

How we mourn is affected by our gender, beliefs, and culture. Men, for example, are not allowed to cry openly as women are. Some cultures encourage public mourning while others prohibit it.

Also, what may cause one to have grief may not cause another. For example, the loss of a child can completely devastate one mother while leaving another seemingly unmoved.

It is important to note that though a person may seem numbed or removed from the grief situation, they could still be grieving. A form of grief is shutting out reality so that you do not have to deal with it.

Mourning is helpful after experiencing a loss. It helps the bereaved make sense of their loss as death is a heavy matter to the heart.

The duration of mourning will vary across families, cultures, personalities, religions and societal norms. These same factors may also determine if a bereaved person is comfortable to seek help. It will also determine the appropriate ways in which friends and relatives can empathize and offer sympathy to the bereaved. Finally, it will also determine how soon the bereaved can move on as some cultures require a family to mourn for a long time.

45. What are the stages of grief?

After experiencing a loss, most people go through a sequence of stages as they grieve. Elisabeth Kubler Ross in her exemplary work outlined five stages of grief. This has now been modified to seven stages. The stages are not meant to neatly package the complex grief process. On the contrary, they are meant to help you navigate the rough terrain of the grief process. Not everyone goes through all these stages. Also, the stages do not have to follow the outlined sequence.

Shock

After receiving the tragic news, whatever it is, one is often thrown into a state of shock and disbelief. Some people may scream or appear to have lost it for some time. Others may just appear awestruck.

Denial

As you struggle to come to grips with the news, you may find yourself wanting to deny it. In the case of a molar diagnosis, you may insist that the doctor carry out another test to confirm if it is indeed true. You may also be convinced that you heard a heartbeat or have a "strong feeling" that the diagnosis could be inaccurate.

Bargaining

As time elapses and reality begins to sink, you may start to bargain with God about the situation. Here, it seems like you are willing to give up something if only it would reverse the situation. You may promise to stop a bad habit if the diagnosis can only be reversed.

Guilt

In this stage, you are coming to term with reality and may start to blame yourself for what happened. You may find yourself analyzing the events leading to perhaps the miscarriage or diagnosis and find ways to blame yourself. Perhaps if I ate a healthier diet or did not expose myself to 123 this would not have happened.

Anger

In this stage, you have accepted things for what they are but have shifted the blame to others. You are angry at God, your partner, the doctor or anyone else who may have contributed in any way to this loss.

Depression

If you do not find help from somewhere, you may find yourself sinking into depression. The emotions of grief and loss are overwhelming and can easily take you down.

Acceptance and hope

With a good support system, you will navigate through the stages of grief successfully until you finally accept and move on. Here you will be able to view the loss positively and be able to plan for another try in the future.

46. How can I tell if I am depressed?

Most times it is difficult to self-diagnose depression. Perhaps because you are not anticipating it, and when it happens you are not in a state to make a diagnosis, unless someone close to you points it out.

Depression usually has a negative tag to it, somewhat associated with psychosis. This makes most people shy away from it. However, according to WHO, 350 million people suffer from depression worldwide. If someone points out to you that you could be suffering from depression, do not feel judged or ashamed. Take it positively and seek help. The following symptoms may point towards depression;

- Loss of interest in daily activities of life
- Not wanting to get out of bed in the morning
- Frequent mood swings
- Feelings of despair
- Lack of appetite or overeating
- Loss of weight unintentionally
- Trouble concentrating on anything
- Fatigue
- Insomnia
- Irritability
- Digestive problems that are not responding to treatment
- Suicidal thoughts

If you have most of these symptoms, you need to seek help from a qualified professional

47. I just don't want to think about it?

People respond differently to the diagnosis of a molar pregnancy. Shutting out is one of the ways to deal with the diagnosis. It could also be a part of the grief process and you may find yourself wanting to talk about it later.

Do not feel condemned or pressured to talk about it if you do not feel like it. However, you still need to find a way to process your emotions in a healthy way. Postponed grief can also lead to complicated grief which is harder to deal with.

Processing through the stages of grief can help you understand your own feelings and which stages most closely applies to you. Then work through your emotions and interpretations of your loss and try to come to terms with it.

48. I don't see it as a big deal, I am perfectly okay!

This is hardly ever true. Even when we feel like we are in control, most times we have not yet dealt with the reality. A molar pregnancy loss is a significant loss, though for sure it impacts on others more than the rest.

Even in the event where a mother wasn't aware that she was expecting and ended up with the miscarriage of a molar, the loss is still significant.

That said, do not feel condemned. Only take the feeling with caution. Do not conclude that you are okay before a significant time has elapsed. Also, the diagnosis of a molar pregnancy leads to many uncertainties such as a subsequent molar and persistent GTD. You may want to talk to a qualified person to help you understand your own feelings and process what is going on.

49. Should I grieve for a baby that wasn't there in the first place?

This depends on how you view a molar pregnancy, and the controversial question as to when life begins. It is a subjective question and it really does depend on how you feel about it.

If you feel the need to grieve, of course, you are entitled to do so. Let no one try to make your loss seem insignificant.

A molar pregnancy presents just like a normal pregnancy and your body will experience symptoms and changes similar to a normal pregnancy. Most significantly, you will not be aware that you are carrying a molar. Therefore, the loss of this pregnancy will be similar to the loss of a normal pregnancy.

Go easy on yourself and feel free to mourn as it comes naturally.

If you do not feel the need to mourn, that is okay too. No one should condemn you. Most women grieve this loss, but it is okay not to do so.

Whether you view the loss of a molar pregnancy as a real loss or not should be up to you.

50. I hadn't told anyone because I wanted it to be a surprise?

This could be devastating and might throw you off at first. It is quite confusing to say, "I was pregnant, but not really pregnant, but now I am not" Uh?

It is much simpler to say that I had a miscarriage, or we lost a pregnancy.

The first thing you need to decide is who you want to share this news with. It needs to be someone who will give you the support and understanding that you require. It is advisable to steer clear of people who may make insensitive remarks about the situation.

That said, it is important to share this devastating news with someone and not keep it to yourself. The journey after the diagnosis of a molar pregnancy needs a lot of support.

Also remember that you were still pregnant, the viability of the pregnancy notwithstanding. Do not feel ashamed to share your story as it may encourage someone else.

51. Help, I am falling apart!

Research has shown that about 40% of people will suffer from anxiety disorder after bereavement. Feelings of guilt can lead to stress and depression which in turn lead to failing health. Eventually, this becomes a cycle that you cannot get out of.

Do not feel alone in this. Neither should you condemn yourself for not being able to "hold it together"

What you need to do it seek help. A trained therapist will equip you with skills to cope with the situation. It may be helpful if you can get in touch with someone who has been through a similar situation.

There are different groups on Facebook and blogs that are exclusive to victims of molar pregnancy; you can get immense support from there too. My molar pregnancy is available as a blog and as a Facebook page. What to expect also has a page dedicated to molar pregnancy. "Molar stories" is also a blog dedicated to molar pregnancy.

Family and friends can also come in to relieve you of duties you may be struggling to handle. Having company will take your mind off the loss and this can also be helpful.

Resist the temptation to self-prescribe pills. In case your situation seems to be getting out of control, kindly seek professional help and inform your doctor.

52. Should I remember this child?

Yes, if you feel the need to, and no, if it will hold you back from "moving on" with life.

It just depends on how healthy your decision is. You may choose to name your lost child and number them among your children. You may choose to keep some memorabilia in their honor.

The underlying motivation is what is critical.

For some, they may see this period as a "depressing memory" and as soon as they are through with mourning, they may want to destroy all memory of it.

For others, they may want to do something to attach meaning to this significant loss.

A complication arises when you hold onto this memory so much so that you fail to move on after the loss. This is called complicated grief and is dealt with below.

53. Why me?

If you are at a place where the question "why me" is constantly on your mind, you are not alone. In the stages of grief outlined by Elisabeth Kubler Ross, she describes this as anger towards God. You may relate this event to other painful situations that you have gone through in the past and try to compare it with the lives of your happy-go-lucky friends. It may seem that bad luck is only directed at you. Worse still, you may feel that you are a better person who does a lot of good and therefore does not deserve this.

These are all normal feelings of grief and you should not feel guilty about having them.

What you need to do is seek help. It may be useful to join online groups, in the absence of physical groups, where you can hear others share their stories. It will be vital for you to know that you are not alone in this and there is a rainbow after the storm.

54. What is complicated grief?

Complicated grief will start out as normal grieving. However, it extends beyond the normal grieving time frame so that you never quite get out of the grieving cycle. Every phase will leave you worse off than the previous one. If you are still intensely grieving six months to one year after your loss, you may be suffering from complicated grief. Some common symptoms of complicated grief include:

- Intense pain and sorrow that lasts over a year
- You are constantly pinning about your loss

- Excessive attachment to reminders of your loss or complete avoidance
- Inability to carry out your usual activities six months to one year after your loss
- Intense bitterness that is prolonged for over six months
- Depression
- Suicidal thoughts
- In general, if you are still having the same intense feelings of grief a year after your loss you may be suffering from complicated grief. This is especially if you are unable to resume most of your daily activities like work and social life. A doctor, psychologist or bereavement counselor will be able to help you deal with complicated grief.

55. What should I do with all the baby stuff I had bought for this child?

There is no one correct answer to this question. What most people have found helpful is to put away the baby stuff for a while as you mourn your loss. Putting them away may help to shorten your grieving period as each time you see the stuff you may be taken back to your loss.

After this period is over, you will be in a better position to decide. Should you be planning to try for another baby, it will be advisable to keep all the stuff, so you do not have to shop again. Remember that you can conceive soon after a molar pregnancy, there is hope.

However, if the baby stuff will bring bad memories, there is no harm in giving the stuff away. You can also ask a close friend to help you sell the stuff, so you can keep the money to be put to some use.

Another idea would be to donate the stuff to a needy baby in memory of your lost child. Some people have found great comfort in doing this, believing that they are doing it in honor of the lost child

Lastly, you could choose to keep a single item as memorabilia, like a vest or sock.

It will be great if you will get to the place where you can view this as a triumph through a difficult situation. So that the memory of it is a positive one.

56. What to do when insensitive remarks are thrown your way?

You should be prepared to hear a couple of insensitive remarks directed at you. This can be very hurtful considering the intense pain you could be going through. The same places where you ran to find comfort become sources of fresh wounds for you.

But the truth is, most people are uninformed about molar pregnancies. So, these remarks may be offered with utmost sincerity and good intention. Chose to see it from this angle.

A few typical insensitive remarks that you may hear include:

- At least it happened early before you bonded with the child

- It was not a real pregnancy so there was no real loss
- Don't worry you will get another child
- At least you have another child
- It happened for the best
- At least you have an angel watching over you
- It could have been worse
- It also happened to so and so

Be selective about who you share this news with. Other than that, just be prepared to hear such remarks and choose to view it as coming from a sincere but uninformed place. So, do not take it to heart.

57. I missed the baby and got cancer instead.

What is most disheartening about a molar pregnancy diagnosis is the cancer possibility that comes with it. Your joy is instantly transformed into fear of the unknown.

In the unfortunate event that you develop persistent gestational trophoblastic disease or choriocarcinoma, do not lose hope.

It may be helpful to join an online support group for moms going through the same experience. Remember that choriocarcinoma is highly curable and that you can still go on to have a healthy pregnancy after receiving treatment.

The tendency is to feel very unfortunate and this may lead you towards depression. So, you need to find support to carry you through this period.

58. What if my partner isn't grieving?

We all grieve in different ways. Also, how we cope with the news of a molar pregnancy will vary from one individual to another. This is dependent on our gender, genetic makeup, socialization, cultural factors or personal experiences.

It is good to discuss it between the two of you openly so that you understand how each person is coping. Remember that there is no right or wrong way to grieve.

The person grieving should not condemn the other or vice versa.

Also, you should avoid judging the other and concluding that they were not interested in the pregnancy.

Talking openly about it will prevent feelings of bitterness from developing between you.

If either of you feels the need to see a therapist as a couple, it may be needful to oblige.

59. For how long should I grieve?

There is no specific amount of time that you are required to grieve. Allow yourself to grieve for as long as you feel the need to. Also, do not feel judged if you grieve for a very short period. If you want to move on as soon as possible it is still okay.

What should alert you is if the grief is prolonged beyond a year after the loss, this could signal complicated grief and will require the attention of a trained professional.

It is not that you are required to completely forget the loss like it never happened, this would be unrealistic. It is that you will be able to move on with your life as it was before after the grieving period is over.

60. Do I want to share my story?

This is okay if it will help in your healing process. You need to decide how much information you want to share and how you want to share it.

Facebook groups could be an easy place to start as you can just post in terms of questions or short posts. But the posts should be exclusive to a molar pregnancy group or a closely related group, otherwise be prepared to listen to a lot of insensitive remarks.

There are also a couple of blogs that have exclusive molar pregnancy sections. You can share your story here too. Additionally, you could answer other people's questions and in that way be of help to them as you share your story.

If you are up to it, you can also start your own blog where you can share your story, offer general information and invite others to share their stories too.

Still, you can write a book about your story.

This list is endless. You could go on national television and other open forums where you can share your story. This can help you heal, encourage another person going through the same situation and help in creating much-needed awareness on the condition.

61. Where can I get support?

You will need a lot of support after the diagnosis of a molar pregnancy.

First, you will need support from your medical team. Do not shy away from seeking help from your doctor whenever you have questions to ask or have clarifications to be made.

Your friends and family can also be very resourceful at this time. They may offer both psychological and practical help to help you get through this phase.

Social groups are also a great resource especially when they include people who have been through the same ordeal. The advantage with such groups is that you are less likely to hear insensitive remarks. But do not compare any one person's story with yours because you may get discouraged if their progress seems faster than yours.

The role of professional therapy cannot be underscored. Talking to a professional will help you better understand your grief and cope with it in a healthy way.

62. What to do when no one understands your grief.

If you are at a place where you feel that no one completely gets you, do not worry, it is okay. The loss of a child is a very personal experience, and no one experiences it the same way as you. Only you know how long you had waited for this baby, how hard you tried or whatever circumstances surround this loss.

There are many paths towards self-healing that you can pursue, it may be lonely, but don't you give up. Be determined to find healing for yourself.

Do not make it your sole ambition to find that person that will resonate 100% with you. Instead, seek healing for yourself because you are the one that needs that healing.

63. How do I move on from here?

Take it one day at a time.

Once you have been cleared by your doctor to try again for another baby and you feel ready to, move on. This may help to psychologically move you to the next phase.

In case you do not want to try again, resume your daily life with more strength and positivity.

Remember that you have just gotten through an experience that would have completely shattered your life, but it didn't. And you came out stronger on the other side.

References

Grief and mourning.com – **Grief and mourning, what's the difference?**

MedicineNet.com – **Loss, grief and bereavement**

Help guide –Coping with grief and loss.

Mental health America –Coping with loss, bereavement and grief

Web MD-What is normal grieving and the stages of grief

Chapter five

For partners

This section is exclusively dedicated to partners/fathers for the unequaled role they play in this journey. They are the forgotten victims of this tragedy. They are the unsung heroes. They are pushed to the sidelines of the action as everyone rushes past them to give sympathy to the mother. Rarely do we stop to ask about the father. True to the words of the poem, he can only break down in the confines of the bathroom and needs to dry his tears before she can see it. He watches her fall asleep before he can allow himself to break down and pour his heart out.

When a couple is expecting, both the mother and father have equal expectation and anticipation of the new life. Both have the expectation of soon becoming parents, or parents again. Though the man's body does not physically change to accommodate this new addition, his heart, emotions, and psychology all tune into fatherhood mode. Therefore, when this dream and desire is cut short, he is as broken as the mother is.

But the man goes through a unique experience in that he is rarely acknowledged as a victim. He is not expected to be breaking down, first because he is a man and 'men don't cry' and because he is expected to be strong for the victim who is the mom.

Indeed, a couple of men will not even expect themselves to be affected in the first place and they will assume that the mom is more vulnerable. For sure it is she who will have to physically go through the "process" but the emotional and psychological drain on both partners cannot be underscored.

If you as a man find yourself wearing this shoe, this chapter is for you. After many long nights of being strong and giving her the support she needs, keeping the family in sync and things running, it may begin to weigh down on you down. As people fade and you are left alone, it slowly sinks in that you feel the loss too. But are you allowed to show weakness? And where can you turn to for help? The following 8 questions will help you explore your own emotions at this time and offer pointers to when you might need professional help.

64. Am I in this?

Yes, you are as much of a victim as the mother is.

The fact that many people may not acknowledge this should not matter. A child has two parents and you are one of them.

It is usual for the mother to seem more affected and as a result attract more sympathy. By their nature, most women are very expressive and will openly show emotion by breaking down, talking, writing etc. and their fellow women are quicker to show sympathy to their counterpart. And of course, the medical team will be more concerned about the mother and what she needs to do after that and how you can support her.

This may leave you feeling left out.

It is okay to acknowledge to yourself that you are also going through significant pain, especially your partner. They may feel comforted in knowing that there is someone equally sharing in their pain and loss.

Do not be afraid to admit to yourself and others that it is equally weighing on you and that you may need support too. Your physical appearance may not have changed in anticipation of fatherhood, but your emotions and psyche were all geared up at this prospect. Meaning your hopes were equally thwarted by the announcement of a molar pregnancy.

65. Was it my fault?

It was not anyone's fault. Neither yours nor hers.

Many risk factors predispose one to molar pregnancy. They include genetics, nutrition, history of a previous molar pregnancy, gestational age among others.

Genetic factors could be linked to either the father or mother. That said, you have no control over genetic factors.

Also having one molar pregnancy does not mean that you cannot get a healthy bay after that. It really is a matter of chance, and luckily enough, the odds are for you.

A better way to look at it instead of trying to apportion blame is being thankful that you can still get healthy babies after a molar pregnancy. This should be an event that draws you closer and does not pull you apart.

66. Why doesn't anyone understand my pain?

Men don't cry

We have heard this so many times or said it ourselves to our fellow men and brothers. We do not allow men to show weakness or emotion.

The loss of a child is one of the most painful experiences one could ever go through. It is very unfair to expect a father to be strong at such a time.

But the truth is, society has primed us not to acknowledge emotional pain in men, even when we can sense it. So, the issue sometimes is that as much as someone may want to offer help, they are not sure how to go about it.

If that is the case, you need to find someone who you can be vulnerable with. Do not assume that everyone is not acknowledging your pain because some do but are just stranded on how to offer help.

 A professional counselor could be of help too as they are more likely to understand your pain.

67. She says that I am unaffected?

Both you and your partner could be very vulnerable at this time. As a result, you may find yourselves up against each other for no apparent reason. Perhaps it's the first time you have been through such a kind of loss together and do not really know how to work through it together. Your ways of grieving may be completely different. You may have silent expectations of each other which when not met will result in frustrations.

It is important to talk freely and support each other through this process. Let her acknowledge that your way of grieving may be different and let her know what you are going through at each time.

Seeing a professional counselor could also be of much help as they may teach you skills to work through the process together.

68. I feel like I am crumbling, is this normal?

It is very normal to feel like you are crumbling, especially if you did not anticipate the impact this loss would have on you.

If you have bottled up your emotions for long and not found an opportunity to deal with the loss, at some later point you will probably crumble.

What you can do is slow down and give yourself some time to grieve your loss. It is okay to let others know what you are feeling and accept the support they offer.

An important person to be vulnerable to is your partner. She needs to be in the know of your emotional and psychological state for her to offer support to you.

However, if you feel like you might be sinking into some form of depression, you should professional help.

The following signs may guide you in self-diagnosing depression; insomnia, constant fatigue, panic attacks, inability to focus for long periods, inability to go on with normal life activities, lack of appetite or overeating and suicidal thoughts.

69. How do I offer her support?

Your partner needs you to be there for them, as much as you need them to be there for you. She will first need you to be physically present to offer a literal shoulder to lean on. She will also need you to be available perhaps to run errands she might not be able to do for herself. She will need you to be available for clinic visits. She will need you to take over mother roles at home that she might not be able to attend to. Emotionally she will need you to be available to connect with her emotionally and be vulnerable with your emotions too. She wants to know your pain and how you are dealing with it. At the same time, she wants you to be strong for her. It is a balancing act.

70. When should I seek professional help?

This is a very important question that cannot be overemphasized.

Men are more likely to suffer from complicated grief than women are. This is because of the unfair expectations society has on men when it comes to showing emotions.

The loss of a child evokes such a strong emotion that is hard to describe. Unfortunately, it is easy for a man to postpone his grief to deal with current high-pressure issues. By the time his grief catches up with him, he is just unable to cope.

Complicated grief in its most basic sense is grief or mourning that extends for more than a year. If after one year you still feel the same strong emotion of loss and pain and are unable to move on with life, you may need to seek professional help.

71. How can I ask for help?

Do not shy away from seeking help and support from those around you. It is unfortunate that there are no online groups exclusive for molar pregnancy dads or such.

That said, there are still adequate resources that you can tap into. Your partner is one of them. Since you are going through this together, being vulnerable with her can help you heal while bringing you closer. Close friends and family can offer both emotional support and be available to relieve you of some duties to give you time to rest.

Professional counseling is also a good option. You may seek counseling individually or as a couple.

Remember that the role you play as a father and partner is a very crucial role. It is important that you are in your best frame to handle this responsibility effectively. Do not shy away from expressing emotion and seeking help when the need arises, in the long run, it will be of benefit to your whole family to have you in your best shape.

For caregivers

I am one myself, and I know what it feels like to find yourself struggling to give appropriate words of comfort to a molar pregnancy patient. When you cannot say, I know what it feels as you are not really sure what it feels like, and the medical textbooks did not adequately prepare you for this time.

This section is not just for healthcare workers, but for every person offering care and support to a molar pregnancy victim. You could be a friend or family member or a therapist or colleague. As long as you are part of the support system of a molar pregnancy victim, this is for you.

The incidence of molar pregnancy is quite low, and you will not hear molar pregnancy being given too much airplay. The awareness is low, and no one will blame you if you hadn't heard of it before it happened to this person now. So, it is understandable to be caught off guard and not know what exact words of encouragement to give.

That said, it is needful to understand the journey and emotional experience of a molar pregnancy victim for you to be able to give them the support they need from you. Having little knowledge will lead to a common pitfall that can be very devastating to the victim, against your intentions. This is insensitive remarks. I have added a list of 10 insensitive remarks and how to avoid them.

The role you play as a caregiver is an important role and cannot be underestimated. If you are equipped with knowledge, you can speed the healing process of the victim.

This section will guide you on how to approach this process, avoid common pitfalls and explore your own emotions around the issue. It contains 7 questions.

72. What is my role in this?

As a caregiver, your role is to offer support in the best way you can to the victims.

You need to be able to empathize with them, offer tangible solutions and alert them when you think they may need extra help. You can also take over their other responsibilities until they are able to do so.

You need to equip yourself with knowledge and basic counseling skills to adequately play this role. You do not need to be a counselor to fit this role, just being able to read cues and encouraging them to express their emotions in a safe space is sufficient.

The truth is, sometimes what they may need is space. You may help by restricting visitors and intruders or yourself moving away for a while to allow them to have that space.

73. What if she has not asked for my help?

Most victims will rarely ask for help directly. Most times, you will have to read cues to decipher what kind of help they may need at that point in time.

If you are close to them, you can easily tell their needs like what responsibilities they may need you to take over, whether they prefer company or want to be left alone.

If it gets to a point where you feel that they may be pushing you away, it is good to take a step back and allow them to breathe. But you may still need to keep checking on them and letting them know that you are available to offer help when needed.

74. What if I am not qualified to give help?

Your role is not to give professional help, there is someone else to do that. But before they even get there, you can play a vital role in their healing process.

Most times, people just like to have someone around to offer company because when they are alone they recall their loss. They need you to be there to hear them vent and express their frustrations to. Rarely will they demand answers from you, unless rhetorical.

That said, you need to be sensitive enough to monitor their grief process. In case you think they are sinking into a depression, you should enlist the help of a qualified professional.

You can offer solutions to common problems such as driving them to the clinic, organizing help around the house and trying to engage them in activities that will uplift their spirits.

Be cautious with your "words of encouragement", sometimes what you speak out of a sincere heart may create deep wounds in how it is interpreted.

75. I feel so much pity?

No one loves being pitied. This portrays your perception of their situation as hopeless and irredeemable. They may, in turn, resent you for it.

What you need to do is to show empathy. Acknowledge the pain that they are going through, allow them to express their emotion without being judgmental and help them work through the grief process.

Do not pretend to know exactly what they are going through unless you have been a victim of molar pregnancy yourself. But even then, your situations cannot be identical.

Also, do not be completely quiet about the situation, as if nothing ever happened. You can ask simple questions such as

- How are you doing emotionally?
- Would you like to talk about how you are feeling?
- Is today better than yesterday?
- Did you eat, sleep, and have a bath?
- What do you feel about your latest hcg readings?
- Do you feel prepared for chemo?

Such open-ended questions will encourage the victim to talk and vent out their emotions. This will help you understand how they are doing, anticipate their needs and offer direction.

Being quiet may make the victim feel like you are undermining their experience or are numb to the pain that they are going through.

Instead of showing pity on them, you can highlight the strength they have exhibited and the progress they are making. This will help them view the situation in a positive light and feel supported by you.

76. Should I encourage her to mourn her loss?

It is not your call to decide whether they need or do not need to mourn. Your role is to offer support in whatever direction they have decided to take.

Most victims will want to mourn their loss but in different ways. There is no correct way to mourn. Some people will talk about it others will not. Some people will be completely devastated others will appear strong. After a few interactions, you will be able to know how the victim has chosen to handle it.

Mourning instantly is usually a good indicator if it is not prolonged beyond six months to a year. When people mourn, they can heal and move on.

Be cautious about a victim who shows no sign of mourning as they may do so later when they should have moved on.

However, some people may show no obvious sign of mourning and ten years later they are still okay. It all depends on one's perception of the event and the coping mechanisms they have built over time.

77. I think she is getting depressed?

As a caregiver, one of the things you need to be on alert for are signs of depression. If you spot these signs, you need to call in extra help to redeem the situation: prolonged insomnia, complete lack of appetite or overeating, inability to focus for a long time, not able to go on with daily activities, avoiding social interactions, being unkempt, too much drinking and dependence on pills, frequent panic attacks, and suicidal thoughts.

Do not ignore such symptoms, especially if they persist for long. As much as it is not easy to point out to someone that they are depressed, in the long run, you will have helped them if they can get help in good time.

78. What are the common pitfalls and how do I avoid them?

The common pitfall we are going to tackle here is insensitive remarks.

Most times, we make insensitive remarks out of a good heart and sincerely wanting to give comfort. The gap is in the knowledge of what molar pregnancy is and what emotional and psychological impact it has on the victims. Some of the common ones include:

- At least the pregnancy was just three months old.
- Your child is always your child from conception. You do not love your teenager any more than you love

your toddler. The moment you realize that you are expecting, an immense love for the child flourishes in your heart.

- There was no baby in the first place
- I am already battling with this news, that there was no viable pregnancy. So, don't rub it in, it doesn't make the pain any less.
- You will get another child
- You do not replace one child with another. I could get ten more, but they will never make up for this one that I lost today.
- It has happened to someone else I know
- The fact that it is 'common' to you does not make it any less painful for me. Tragedy is personal.
- At least you have another/other children
- True I will return home to some happiness, but the pain of this loss cannot be consoled by that fact.
- Now you have an angel watching over you
- I do not need a guardian angel, I want a baby to hold and care for.
- It is for the best
- Then show me what worst would look like? The loss of life and the pain it brings cannot be for the best.
- At least you didn't get to him/her then have them snatched away
- Whether you held your baby in your arms or in your mind, this baby is real to you, and you got to know them and love them unconditionally.
- I know exactly how you feel
- Tell me what I feel? Even if you have been through a molar pregnancy experience yourself, chances are

that your circumstances were different. More so, we all grieve differently.

- Did you do something that you were not supposed to do
- Are you trying to blame me for killing my own baby? That is exactly what it sounds like to me.
- Be grateful that you are still alive
- Honestly, at this point, I'd rather be dead. What is the point in life when it is so unbearable?

Remember that any woman of reproductive age can be a victim of molar pregnancy. The role you are playing today, you may need someone to play it for you in the future.

Developing skills such as empathizing and active listening will make you a better caregiver.

Without knowledge, you may say comments that are more hurtful than if you said nothing in the first place.

References

Family caregiver association – **Care giving 101**

ASCO Cancer.net- **Caring for a loved one**

Matrix Care- **What being a care giver means**

Chapter Six

Finding hope and moving on

Most people are not aware of molar pregnancies. As a result, there is not much support afforded to molar pregnancy victims.

Losing a pregnancy can be devastating, especially when you do not have a strong support system to fall back on. For most women, this is a period of intense pain and confusion because nothing quite prepares you for it. You may feel as if your whole world is caving in and that you have lost a part of yourself.

Shock, anger, emptiness, and yearning for a bay to hold are feelings that you may experience. It is made worse by the fact that despite experiencing a loss of life, there is nothing tangible to mourn over.

It is important for you to grieve so that you will be able to move on after accepting your loss.

Tips to help you recover

Acknowledge your pain

The first step towards healing is accepting what has happened. Admit to yourself that you have lost a pregnancy through a molar pregnancy and that you will not be receiving that child. Also, admit to yourself the pain and heartache that it has caused you. If friends and family try to diminish your pain, do not get disheartened. It is up to you to decide how to mourn your loss.

Allow yourself to grieve

Grieving allows you to let go of the connection you had to the pregnancy and your baby. It allows your heart to release the pain and brokenness. Crying and other ways of mourning have a way of making you heal faster. Pain that is bound up in your heart without expression may stay there for years.

There is no correct or incorrect duration to grieve, allow yourself to let your emotions flow as they come. It may take a month or even up to one year and even after then, the pain may never quite disappear, it just resurfaces less often.

Do something in memory of your lost child

This could be something as simple as planting a flower that will help to give you closure. It helps to feel that you have done something in memory of the child you never got to hold. You could get a mug printed with the name you had chosen for them, you could start a molar pregnancy blog to encourage other mothers going through a similar experience, you could plant a tree or take a hike. Just anything special that has meaning to you, in memory of this child.

Allow your partner to grieve in a different way

One of the most frustrating things to deal with during this period is conflict with your partner. Most times, you are tempted to project the anger and bitterness you have to the person closest to you, who may be your partner. And one of the ways this anger comes out is getting frustrated at their grieving process which may be different from yours.

Remember that you are equal partners in this process. He is hurting as much as you are hurting, only that he may grieve in a much different way from yours.

You may have bonded more with the pregnancy because your body was physically transformed by the changes. But emotionally and psychologically, he experienced his own changes.

How we grieve is affected by so many factors. Giving each other space to grieve in your own way will help you recover faster. Remember that different does not mean better or worse. Talking about your individual process of grief can also be very helpful.

Try to find meaning in your loss

This does not mean trying to undermine your pain or justify your loss. It means acknowledging it as a pain and finding comfort through it. Living through this experience may make you a stronger person; you may discover strength and endurance you did not know existed before. You can be a source of encouragement to someone going through a similar experience in the future.

Be prepared for difficult days

Even after you have healed, some unexpected things may remind you of your loss and take you back emotionally to your pain. Some of the subtle reminders could be like seeing a new-born, hearing a baby's cry, seeing baby items, when your first period resumes or when it gets to your 'would have been' due date.

You can prepare yourself psychologically on how to handle such situations; you can plan to be with someone or plan to avoid the situations if you can.

Find a support network

Build a strong support network to carry you through at least the first year of your loss. An important group is people who have been through a similar situation. Thankfully, there are a couple of social media groups and blogs that are exclusive to molar pregnancy victims. Your immediate family and friends can also offer you support. When helps comes your way, do not turn it down.

See a therapist

If you feel stranded at any one point, seek professional help. A trained counselor or psychologist will equip you with coping skills to get you through this difficult phase.

Read literature that will uplift you

You must remain positive by saturating yourself with positive thoughts. Read about hopeful situations. Read books on molar pregnancy and stories of people who have lived through the experience and have success stories. You must push yourself to find hope beyond the molar pregnancy. If you desire to have another baby, read about people who have conceived after molar pregnancies. It is advisable to keep a positive attitude so that you do not sink into fear and depression.

Take a vacation

If you can afford, take a vacation. It can be a budget or a luxury break. Time away will help you refocus your energies and heal. Take a break from people who may ask you many questions and intrude your space so that by the time you get back, you are ready to deal with your new reality.

Eat healthily and exercise

Do not neglect your body. Food goes a long way in determining your mood. You are more likely to feel depressed when you are not on a healthy diet.

Your body also needs to recover physically after the process of a molar pregnancy. Eating a well-balanced diet and using supplements can put you in a better shape. This will help you heal and move on.

Purpose to get through this

It is important that you desire to heal and get through the experience positively. As hard as it may seem, keep your mind focused on a positive end where you are healed. Healing does not mean completely forgetting about the experience, it means that the experience does not cause as much pain and that despite the pain, you are able to carry on with life.

At the end of the day, life must go on. Pain is an integral part of everyone's life. Pain should not break us but make us stronger.

Breaking the silence about molar pregnancy.

Why is awareness important?

When you speak up, you allow many other voices to echo you.

Molar pregnancy has been in the closets for long enough. We speak about it in hushed tones and as a result, victims feel embarrassed, abnormal and secluded. The mystery surrounding molar pregnancy has made it difficult for victims to seek help openly.

When we create awareness, we will help create better support systems for the victims starting from equipped health personnel, equipped hospitals, increased research and increased funding for molar pregnancy.

Ways to create awareness

Storytelling

Stories could be told through various channels. A simple one is social media groups where victims can share their experiences with other victims. Blogs are also effective and there are already a couple of blogs doing this. Radio and TV interviews are rare but also a good opportunity when the chance presents itself. These are very good and have a wider coverage. Books are also another good way to share stories. The book can be in e form or print form.

Awareness walks, marathons, and hikes

This is good for creating mass awareness and may attract the government's eye and trigger government action. Funds collected could go into a molar pregnancy kitty to fund research and such activities that may help in a greater cause.

Having small group talks

Creating talks on molar pregnancy in small groups to sensitize women on risk factors for molar pregnancy. Target groups are groups with women of reproductive age. The focus should just be on creating awareness remembering that one in a thousand women is likely to develop a molar pregnancy.

What next from here?

You have gotten through the ups and downs of a molar pregnancy and now you are at the other end. So, what's next?

Trying again for a rainbow baby

In case you are considering having another baby, you should start getting excited about it.

This is not to say that trying again will be easy. It may be harder on you emotionally seeing what you have been through. It can be an emotional roller coaster as you swing between excitement, anxiety, hope, and paranoia.

But you should know that chances of another molar pregnancy are still minimal, 1/68. Also, your fertility is unaffected by the molar pregnancy. So, you are starting at the same place as any other woman, not at a harder place physiologically.

View the molar pregnancy as a single isolated event that speaks nothing of your chances of getting a healthy baby. Consider that many women have gone ahead to get healthy babies soon after. Actually, some have conceived sooner after the molar than before.

If you are planning on trying to conceive after experiencing a miscarriage, here are some tips to help you:

Study your cycle

You have probably heard that women ovulate on the 14th day of their cycle, which is inaccurate. The 14th day is just an estimation of the middle of your menstrual cycle.

Studying your cycle will help you know the right days to have intercourse that you are more likely to conceive. There are two methods you can use to study your cycle: charting and studying your body for ovulation changes naturally. Charting is effective but may be tiresome for many. Using charting kits may take away from the natural process of trying to conceive.

Alternatively, these 10 signs can guide you in telling if you are ovulating.

- Increased cervical mucus, the color will be egg white and the texture will be slippery between your fingers.
- You may have a heightened sex drive, luckily. Perhaps it is nature's way of ensuring the furtherance of the reproduction agenda.
- Increased breast tenderness.
- Slight increase in weight. Your clothes may fit a bit more tightly. This is due to increased water retention.
- Bloating.
- Your vaginal lips may swell and be tender to touch.
- Slight cramping referred to as mittelschmerz.
- Less occasionally, you may have a mood boost
- Some women experience ovulation spotting
- Some women experience headaches and nausea.

You can try to lengthen your luteal phase

The luteal phase is the second half of your cycle, the time from after you ovulate to the first day of the next cycle. A typical luteal phase will range from 12 to 14 days, but it really is unique for each woman. A luteal phase that is shorter than 12 days should be a concern.

If your luteal phase is shorter than 12 days your body may not be producing enough progesterone to support a pregnancy. Progesterone is vital for a healthy pregnancy. It first helps in the thickening of the uterus lining to make it ready for implantation. It also helps the cervix to form the mucus plug on the cervical opening that will protect the developing baby from infection.

A couple of natural supplements are geared towards lengthening your menstrual cycle. Vitex, red raspberry leaf and vitamin B6 are some of them.

Eat a healthy diet and take care of yourself.

Make sure your body is in great shape and form emotionally physically and psychologically. Feed well and exercise. Being malnourished has a negative impact on your fertility.

Take folic acid, kick off alcohol and cigarettes and limit caffeine intake.

Take a baby making break

Occasionally, after you have tried for a while with no success, take a break to rejuvenate and release the stress.

Enjoy your sex life just for the physical pleasure and stop obsessing about the baby for a while.

Consult a fertility specialist

If you have been trying for very long with no success, it is best to seek specialist help. For women aged 35 and younger, very long is up to one year. For women aged over 35, seek help after trying for six months.

Certain conditions may also affect your fertility. It is better to seek treatment if you have any of these conditions, otherwise, you may keep trying with no success. They are fibroids, endometriosis, pelvic inflammatory disease, polycystic ovarian syndrome, STDs, blocked fallopian tubes and chronic illnesses such as diabetes, cancer and thyroid disease.

Side note

If you choose not to try again for a baby, it should not be because of fearing that you will go through the ordeal again. Because if fear is your motivator, chances are that you have not healed completely. You may want to talk to a qualified counselor or psychologist.

Do not lose hope!

114

One last thing… In the spirit of raising awareness, I would like to ask you to leave an honest review about this book on Amazon. It really does make a big difference.

I also want to give you a chance to win a **$200.00 Amazon Gift Card** as a thank-you for reading this book.

All I ask is that you give me some feedback! You can also copy/paste your *Amazon* or *Goodreads review* and this will also count.

Your opinion is valuable to me. It will only take a minute of your time to let me know what you like and what you didn't like about this book. The hardest part is deciding how to spend the two hundred dollars! Just follow this link.

http://reviewers.win/molar

References

Miscarriage association- Trying again

American pregnancy association – Getting pregnant again, after a miscarriage

WebMD- Am I ovulating?

NHS Choices – How can I tell if I'm ovulating?

Resourceful molar pregnancy links

My molar pregnancy.com

Baby centre community – **Molar and partial molar pregnancy**

Molar pregnancy support and information

Molar stories blog

My molar pregnancy.com **Facebook page**

Baby and bump – **Molar and partial molar support group.**

Web MD – **Molar pregnancy**

American pregnancy – **Molar pregnancy**

Tommy's – **Molar stories**